"A Comprehensive and Insightful Guide to the World of Stem Cell Therapy"

"Stem Cell Therapy in a Nutshell" is an outstanding resource that bridges the gap between complex scientific research and practical clinical application. It provides a comprehensive understanding of the potential and limitations of stem cell therapy, making it an essential read for anyone involved in or considering this innovative treatment approach. As a practitioner, I highly recommend this book to my colleagues and patients alike, confident that it will enhance their knowledge and appreciation of the remarkable capabilities of stem cell therapy."

—Dr. Sunny Kim, MD Specialist in Regenerative Medicine, President and CEO, Progressive Regenerative Medicine Clinic, PC; Founder, GenXovite Global Think Tank

"The book serves as an indispensable and comprehensive resource for anyone looking to delve into the world of stem cell therapy. It offers a thorough introduction to the science, applications, and ethical considerations surrounding stem cells, making it an essential read for healthcare professionals. I highly recommend this guide to all doctors who are incorporating stem cells into their practice. It provides the foundational knowledge needed to understand the potential and limitations of this powerful therapeutic tool."

—Dr. Dennis Harper, DC, ND, Regenerative Clinic Owner and Founder of Harper Restoration Systems

"Stem Cell Therapy in a Nutshell" by Dr. Hans-Thomas Richter is an insightful and accessible guide to the rapidly evolving field of regenerative medicine. This book expertly bridges the gap between complex scientific research and practical clinical applications, providing a thorough understanding of stem cell therapies, particularly mesenchymal stem cells (MSCs), and their potential in treating various conditions.

Dr. Richter demystifies the science, explores ethical considerations, and discusses both the promise and limitations of stem cell therapies. Drawing on decades of experience, he offers valuable insights for healthcare professionals, researchers, and patients alike. "Stem Cell Therapy in a Nutshell" is a must-read for anyone interested in the future of medicine and the transformative possibilities of stem cell research.

Kitsap Publishing is proud to present this comprehensive and enlightening resource, essential for navigating the complex landscape of modern healthcare.

—**Reprospace Editorial Reviews™**

Stem Cell Therapy in a Nutshell

Demystifying Stem Cells

Hans-Thomas Richter, Ph.D., MAcOM

Stem Cells in a Nutshell
First Edition 2024

By Dr. Hans-Thomas Richter

Paperback ISBN-978-1-952685-88-0

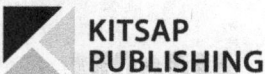

KITSAP PUBLISHING

Published by Kitsap Publishing
Poulsbo, WA 98370
www.KitsapPublishing.com

Contents

Dedication

To the countless patients, many of whom I treated in my practice over the years, and their families who seek hope and healing through the possibilities of regenerative medicine, your courage, and resilience inspire us to expand the horizons of science every day.

To the researchers, doctors, and healthcare professionals who tirelessly work to transform stem cell science from theory to practice. I dedicate this book to your unwavering commitment to advancing medicine for the betterment of humanity.

And to my own family and friends, whose support and encouragement have been the foundation of this journey—thank you for believing in the power of discovery and the pursuit of knowledge.

May this book not only serve as a guide and a source of hope, but also as a reminder of the remarkable potential within us all to heal and regenerate. Let it inspire us to continue our quest for knowledge and discovery.

Foreword

At Kitsap Publishing, we have always been committed to bringing readers insightful and transformative books on health, alternative medicine, and nutrition. Our mission is to empower individuals to take charge of their well-being through knowledge and informed choices. "Stem Cell Therapy in a Nutshell" by Dr. Hans-Thomas Richter is a valuable addition to our collection, offering a comprehensive and accessible exploration of one of the most promising fields in modern medicine.

Dr. Richter's book delves into the science of stem cells with clarity and depth, making complex concepts understandable for healthcare professionals and laypeople alike. He takes readers on a journey through the different types of stem cells, particularly mesenchymal stem cells (MSCs), and their applications in regenerative medicine. The book provides a balanced view, highlighting both the remarkable potential and current limitations of stem cell therapies.

What sets this book apart is its focus on a paradigm shift in medicine—from a model that often relies on drugs and surgeries to "fix" the body, to one that harnesses the body's natural ability to heal itself. Stem cell therapy represents this shift by promoting regeneration rather than merely managing symptoms. Instead of replacing damaged tissues with artificial materials or suppressing symptoms with medications, stem cell therapy encourages the body to use its innate regenerative powers. This approach not only aligns with more holistic views of health but also offers a gentler, less invasive alternative to traditional treatments.

Kitsap Publishing supports books like "Stem Cell Therapy in a Nutshell" because we believe in the importance of providing access to diverse perspectives on health. Our catalog includes works on integrative medicine, nutrition, and holistic health approaches, reflecting our commitment to empowering readers with the knowledge they need to make informed health decisions. Books like this one challenge conventional thinking and open up new possibilities for healing and wellness.

With decades of clinical experience and scientific research, Dr. Richter provides readers with valuable insights into the current state and future potential of stem cell therapies. This book is an essential resource for anyone interested in exploring the transformative possibilities of regenerative medicine, whether you are a healthcare provider, researcher, or patient.

We are proud to present this book and hope it inspires you to consider new approaches to health and healing. At Kitsap Publishing, we believe that the future of medicine lies in understanding and harnessing the body's remarkable capacity to heal itself. "Stem Cell Therapy in a Nutshell" is a significant step toward realizing that future.

Sincerely,

Ingemar Anderson

Publisher, Kitsap Publishing, Poulsbo, WA

Introduction

"If the Sea of Marrow is abundant, vitality is good, the body feels light and agile, and the span of life will be long."

-The NeiJing, 黃帝內經

As we will discuss this quote in detail later, we welcome you to a journey through the fascinating and rapidly evolving world of "stem cell" therapies. This book is designed as a guide to help you, the reader, navigate the complexities and understand the current landscape of treatments and innovations in this field. The book is not an exhaustive scientific review, rather the author's goal is to demystify the science behind "stem cells" and provide the reader with a clearer picture of what are the possibilities in modern stem cell therapy.

In these pages, we will explore the various types of stem cells – from mesenchymal stem cells found in umbilical cord tissue to the induced pluripotent stem cells created in laboratories. We will delve into their unique characteristics, how they are being used in medicine today, and what future therapies might look like.

My journey into the field of science began early in my career as a student. While pursuing my master's diploma in biochemistry in 1991, I embarked on a research project at the University of Southern California, focusing on chondrogenic fibroblasts. Our goal was to identify the DNA methylation factors that could activate the differentiation process of these cells. This early exposure to stem cell research ignited my passion for understanding the mechanisms of cellular differentiation and regeneration.

More than 30 years later, the world of stem cell therapy is one of immense potential and promise, but it is also a field fraught with complexities and challenges. As a reader seeking to understand this landscape, perhaps as a candidate considering stem cell therapy, it is crucial to have a clear and balanced view of both the potential and the limitations of current treatments. This book aims to equip you with the knowledge and tools to make informed decisions about your health and medical options.

We will also address some of the common misconceptions and ethical considerations surrounding stem cell therapy. It is important to separate fact from fiction, especially in a field that is often sensationalized in the media.

Throughout this book, we will present clinical and research studies, review case studies, and examine the outcomes of various treatments. While the scientific community continues to conduct research and clinical trials, it is our hope that this book will serve as a helpful resource for those interested in understanding the current state of stem cell therapies and what they have to offer.

As you turn these pages, keep in mind that the field of stem cell therapy is continuously evolving. What we know today might just be the tip of the iceberg of what we will discover tomorrow. This book is a snapshot of where we currently stand, a guide to help you understand and navigate the exciting potential of these therapies.

Welcome to your exploration of the world of stem cells – a world where science meets hope, and where the future of medicine is being written one discovery at a time.

Diving deeper into this book, it's important to acknowledge the vast clinical experience accumulated over the past decades, during which several million patients worldwide have undergone various forms of stem cell therapies. This extensive clinical practice has been instrumental in refining our understanding of these therapies, allowing clinics and medical professionals to better evaluate outcomes, set realistic expectations, and continually improve treatment protocols.

The journey of stem cell therapy is not just about the cells themselves, but also about the comprehensive approach to patient care. Clinics worldwide have learned invaluable lessons from each patient treated. This has led to the development of more sophisticated strategies in both the application of stem cell therapies and the crucial post-treatment care. The evolution of these treatments is a testament to the commitment of the medical community to enhance patient well-being and to push the boundaries of regenerative medicine.

Moreover, the integration of adjunct therapies has played a significant role in maximizing the benefits of stem cell treatments. These additional therapies, ranging from nutritional support and physiotherapy to advanced biotechnologies, are tailored to complement stem cell treatments, ensuring that patients receive holistic care. This multifaceted approach underscores the importance of viewing stem cell therapy not in isolation but as part of a broader, more integrated treatment strategy.

The experiences and insights gained from treating such a vast number of patients have also been pivotal in shaping guidelines, standardizing protocols, and setting benchmarks for success. These developments have not only enhanced the safety and efficacy of treatments but have also provided valuable data that drives ongoing research and innovation.

As we explore these themes throughout the book, we will also look into the real stories of patients and clinicians, their challenges, successes, and the lessons learned along the way. These narratives are more than just anecdotes; they are the real-life experiences that shape our understanding and pave the way for future advancements.

Navigating the Complexities of Stem Cell Science

As we dive into the world of stem cell research and therapy, it's important to acknowledge from the outset that this field is marked by its complexity and diversity. In this book, we aim to shed light on this intricate landscape, but it's crucial for readers to bear in mind the inherent challenges and nuances that characterize stem cell science.

Variability in Stem Cell Sources:

One of the fundamental complexities of stem cell research is the variability in cell sources. Stem cells can be derived from various tissues, including adipose (fat), bone marrow, and umbilical cord, among others. Each source carries unique characteristics and potential therapeutic applications, making direct comparisons between them challenging.

Diverse Manufacturing Processes:

Adding to this complexity is the variety of manufacturing processes used in preparing stem cells for clinical use. Different methods of isolation, cultivation, and storage can significantly affect the cells' properties and performance in therapeutic applications.

Heterogeneity in Research Studies: The field is characterized by a multitude of studies, many of which are small-scale due to limited funding. This can lead to a lack of standardization in methodologies and outcomes, making it difficult to compare and contrast study results across different research projects.

Efforts in Characterization:

Researchers are increasingly recognizing the need to precisely characterize stem cell samples. This involves detailing specific markers, such as CD markers, and employing techniques like proteomics to understand the protein compositions of the cells. These efforts are crucial for ensuring consistency and reliability in research findings.

Challenges in Data Comparison:

The heterogeneity in stem cell sources, manufacturing processes, and characterization methods often results in difficulties when attempting to compare data and draw broad conclusions. This aspect is a significant challenge in the field and can sometimes lead to overlooking the nuances of individual studies.

Importance of Quality Control:

Quality control is paramount in stem cell research and therapy. The source and handling of stem cells have profound implications for their efficacy and safety in clinical applications. It is essential to consider these factors when evaluating scientific studies and their outcomes.

Acknowledging the Limitations:

While stem cell research holds tremendous promise, it's also essential to recognize its current limitations. The field is continuously evolving, and what we understand today may be significantly enhanced or modified by future discoveries.

Approaching with a Critical Eye:

As a reader or potential candidate for stem cell therapy, approaching the subject with a critical and informed perspective is crucial. Understanding the source, quality, and handling of stem cells used in any study or therapy is key to making informed decisions. And finally in the appendix you will find information on non-stem cell treatments such as PRP.

In this book, we will delve into these complexities, providing a clearer understanding of the current state of stem cell science and therapy. We will explore the nuances of different stem cell types, the intricacies of their extraction and use, and the challenges and successes of ongoing research. By the end, you should have a more informed view of this dynamic and rapidly advancing field.

In sum, this book seeks to provide a concise view of the current state of stem cell therapy, enriched by decades of clinical practice and patient experiences. As you navigate through the chapters, keep in mind the dynamic nature of this field - a realm where patient care continually evolves, and where each treatment contributes to the broader tapestry of scientific progress and human health.

As to the quote of Albert Einstein "If we knew what it was we were doing, it would not be called research, would it?"- Medicine is largely an empirical science. You just can't argue with properly done statistical results of a medical study outcome. Science and Research studies have to be verified in multiple clinical and peer reviewed study results. They can only guide us towards a better Medicine that benefits all provided that bias can be removed as much as possible. To achieve this goal, we should make sure that there is a collaboration of scientists and clinicians to further this field of Regenerative Medicine and they understand each other's contributions.

Incorporating ancient Wisdom in modern Science

Lastly, we will emphasize the crucial role MSCs play in reducing inflammation and minimizing scar formation, two key factors in regenerative medicine. The latter part explores the quantum biology perspective, examining how fundamental processes at the molecular level, such as the role of docosahexaenoic acid (DHA) in neural cell signaling, contribute to the extraordinary regenerative capabilities of stem cells. Additionally, this part includes a discussion on the ancient wisdom of Traditional Chinese Medicine (TCM) and its concept of essence (Jing), drawing parallels between these traditional views and modern stem cell research. This comprehensive overview provides a deeper understanding of the mechanisms and therapeutic potential of MSCs while integrating historical and contemporary insights.

Disclaimer Notice

None of the statements in this book are FDA approved, and it is unlikely they ever will be. Due to copyright restrictions, we are unable to reproduce many of the beautiful illustrations from various publications. Please refer to the citations provided and review the published peer-reviewed articles separately for detailed information. The author has made every effort to give proper credit to the original authors through the citations included herein.

Part I

Introduction and Basics

Introduction to Stem Cell Therapy Overview and Importance

The emergence of regenerative medicine, particularly stem cell therapy, has set the stage for a paradigm shift in healthcare, offering an alternative to traditional approaches that largely focus on symptom management and surgical intervention. Traditional medicine has primarily been reactive, addressing symptoms and diseases as they occur. It employs a wide array of pharmaceuticals and surgical procedures to manage conditions, providing often essential but temporary relief. Although these treatments can be life-saving and alleviate suffering, they usually don't address the root cause of the condition and may come with various side effects.

In contrast, regenerative medicine focuses on restoring the normal function of organs and tissues that have been damaged due to age, trauma, or disease. Stem cell therapy, a cornerstone of regenerative medicine, aims to replace or repair damaged cells and tissues at the cellular level. This is an inherently proactive approach that seeks to cure the underlying condition rather than merely treating the symptoms. By harnessing the body's innate ability to heal and regenerate, these therapies offer the possibility of longer-lasting and more complete recovery.

The implications of this shift are profound. While traditional treatments like chemotherapy attempt to kill "unhealthy" cells, they also damage healthy cells, leading to debilitating side effects. Stem cell-based treatments could target malignancies more precisely and spur the growth of healthy tissue, offering a less toxic and more effective treatment. Similarly, instead of relying on organ transplants, which come with the risk of rejection and lifelong immunosuppressive medication, regenerative medicine offers the potential to grow new, patient-specific organs in the lab.

Moreover, the economic and social impact of regenerative medicine could be revolutionary. Chronic conditions that require lifetime medication or frequent surgical interventions strain healthcare systems and compromise the quality of life for patients. Regenerative therapies could offer one-time, curative treatments that eliminate the need for ongoing care. This not only would be a more humane approach but could also dramatically reduce healthcare costs in the long term.

In summary, the potential of stem cell therapy offering unique advantages and other regenerative strategies to 'cure' rather than manage conditions is a game-changer. As these treatments become more refined and accessible, they are set to redefine our understanding of 'healthcare', pushing the boundaries from symptom management to actual healing.

The body has an innate ability to regenerate

Indeed, the body's innate healing mechanisms are essentially what truly facilitate recovery, even when traditional Western medical techniques such as surgery and pharmaceuticals are employed. For example, after surgical intervention, it is ultimately the body's own regenerative capabilities—driven largely by stem cells—that promote healing and tissue repair. However, this natural process is not without its drawbacks. One of the main issues with natural tissue repair is the formation of scar tissue, which is essentially a non-functional tissue formed during the healing process. Scar tissue can be counterproductive because it lacks the specialized features of the tissue it replaces, often leading to impaired function.

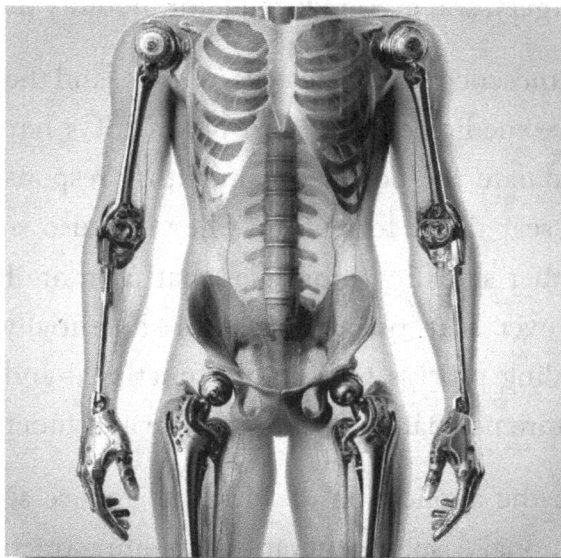

Fig.1: Schematic of a human with artificially replaced bones and joints. Regenerative Medicine hardly gets a chance!

The allopathic approach to decayed or non-functional joints is to replace them with artificial metal. This not only is irreversible and does not give the body a chance to regenerate but it comes with many side effects and new health risks. Any surgery produces more scar tissue and reduces mobility. Furthermore, often there is a need to treat artificial joints with stem cell therapy to counteract the inflammation and scar tissue produced by the surgery.

Scar tissue formation is particularly problematic because the human body does not have an efficient way of reducing or remodeling it once it has formed. Traditional surgical and pharmaceutical interventions have limitations when it comes to preventing or reducing scar tissue. In many cases, surgery can actually exacerbate scar tissue formation, and drugs might not offer a targeted solution for this specific issue. This is a significant concern in numerous conditions, from cardiac fibrosis following a heart attack to adhesions after abdominal surgery, and even reduced joint mobility due to scarring.

This is where mesenchymal stem cells (MSCs) and the broader field of regenerative medicine come into play. MSCs have the unique ability to modulate the body's inflammatory response, which is a key driver of scar tissue formation. They can also secrete growth factors and other signaling molecules that promote healthy tissue regeneration over scar tissue formation. Essentially, MSCs can guide the healing process to be more functional and less fibrotic, aiming to restore normal tissue architecture and function.

Research into the application of MSCs to reduce scar tissue and promote functional tissue regeneration is gaining traction in the scientific community. Clinical studies have shown promising results in applications ranging from reducing corneal scarring to improving outcomes in liver cirrhosis and even spinal cord injuries. As our understanding of MSCs grows, so does the potential to revolutionize how we approach tissue repair and healing post-intervention.

[PMID34359898] It is the non-functional scar tissue resulting for improper repair after trauma that often prohibits healing!

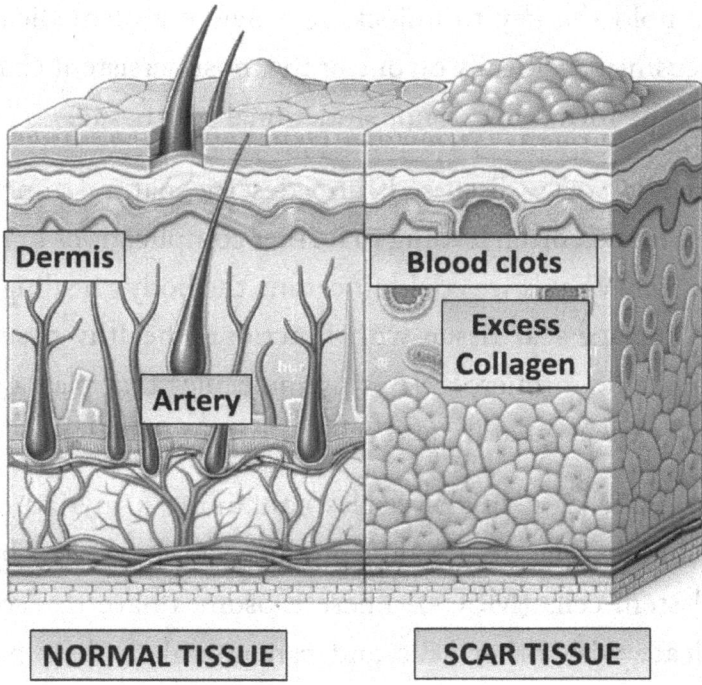

Fig.2: Schematic of the non-functional scar tissues resulting from trauma, interfering with the proper healing process.

In conclusion, while our bodies have a remarkable ability to heal and regenerate, the natural processes at work are not perfect and often result in the formation of problematic scar tissue. The targeted use of MSCs in regenerative medicine offers a promising avenue to correct this shortcoming, actively guiding the healing process away from scar tissue formation and toward the regeneration of functional tissue. This represents not just an incremental improvement over existing medical treatments, but a paradigm shift in our approach to healing and tissue repair.

In the following chapters, we will delve deeper into one of the most fascinating aspects of regenerative medicine— the role of microRNA contained within exosomes. These small but powerful molecules hold the key to unlocking a new era of medical treatments, focusing specifically on one of the most persistent challenges in healing: the formation of non-functional scar tissue.

Scar tissue, as we've discussed, impedes the natural function of organs and tissues, often leading to further complications or reduced quality of life. What if we could fine-tune the body's healing mechanisms to replace scar tissue with functional, healthy tissue? The answer might lie in microRNA, tiny molecules that play a significant role in gene regulation and cellular communication.

Exosomes, which are small vesicles containing a myriad of molecules including microRNA, are produced and released by mesenchymal stem cells (MSCs). These exosomes have the ability to communicate with other cells and can modulate their behavior. Recent research suggests that the microRNA within these exosomes can specifically target and reduce the formation of fibrotic, non-functional tissue, enabling the body to heal in a more effective and functional manner. [PMID35073970]

As we explore the science behind exosomal microRNA, we will take you through the current research landscape, clinical applications, and future prospects of this exciting field. We will also look at case studies where this groundbreaking approach is being applied to improve patient outcomes in conditions ranging from heart disease to liver fibrosis and beyond.

Stay tuned as we navigate through this cutting-edge topic, demystifying the complex mechanisms and showcasing how the next frontier in regenerative medicine could transform the way we understand and approach healing and tissue repair.

This introduction aims to set the stage for the in-depth exploration that will follow, providing readers with an exciting preview of what's to come.

Age-related decline in Stem Cells

As we will discuss extensively later on, the age-related decline in stem cells is a major factor in the aging process and the body's diminished ability to heal. Research by Caplan in 2009 showed that a newborn has up to 200 times more active stem cells in their body compared to an elderly individual. This significant reduction in stem cell activity with age contributes to the decreased regenerative capacity and increased susceptibility to diseases and injuries observed in older adults.

Grouped by decade, a dramatic decrease in MSCs per nucleated marrow cell can be observed:

- Birth to Teens: There is a 10-fold decrease in MSCs, reflecting the rapid decline in stem cell availability as the body transitions from infancy to adolescence.

- Teens to Elderly: Another 10-fold decrease occurs, demonstrating a continued significant drop in MSC numbers into old age.

Impact on Healing

These decreases in MSCs correlate closely with observed fracture healing rates:

- Young Individuals: Healing is very rapid, supported by a high number of MSCs.

- Older Patients: Healing is much slower due to the drastically reduced number of MSCs.

Comparison with HSCs: In contrast, the titres of hematopoietic stem cells (HSCs) in marrow remain constant throughout life, at about one per 10,000 nucleated marrow cells. This stability in HSC levels underscores the unique and critical decline in MSCs as a key factor in age-related regenerative capacity.

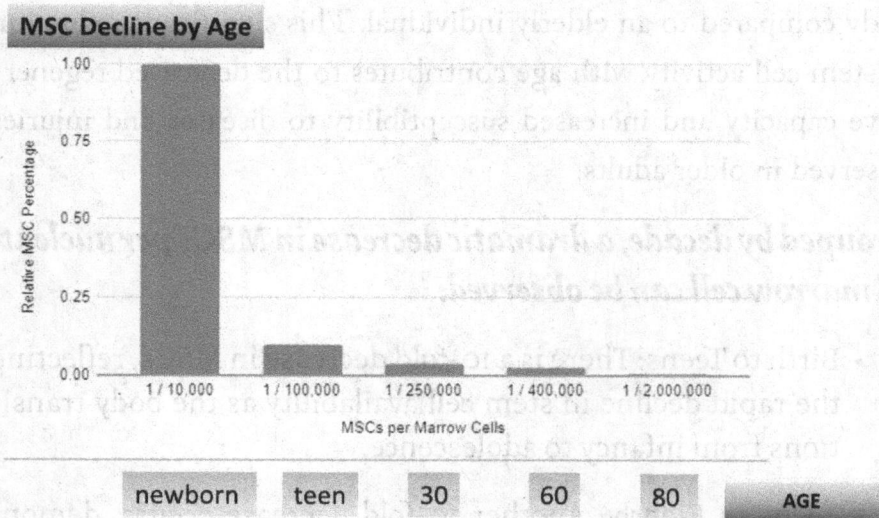

Fig. 3: The decline of Stem cells with age (Marrow MSCs determined by CFU and age): These numbers illustrate the significant reduction as humans age, highlighting the challenges in using autologous MSCs from older patients for regenerative therapies. [adopted from Caplan 2009; PMID19023885]

Understanding this decline is crucial for developing strategies to enhance stem cell function and improve health outcomes across the lifespan. This knowledge paves the way for innovative therapies aimed at mitigating the effects of aging and enhancing the body's natural healing processes.

In 2009 Caplan et. al. [PMID19023885] analyzed the colony forming units (CFU) of Bone Marrow MSCs with age (Fig. 3). These studies have demonstrated that MSCs from older individuals show a decline in proliferation and differentiation potential compared to those from younger individuals. This age-related decline impacts their therapeutic efficacy and is crucial for understanding their use in clinical applications of autologous stem cells.

What is an MSC?

The Medicinal Signaling Cell

Definition and Characteristics

It is important to distinguish MSCs from totipotent or fetal 'stem cells'. They have little in common. In addition, there is some debate of what MSC actually means. Three most common full forms of the abbreviation are:

- Mesenchymal stem cells
- Mesenchymal stromal cells
- Medicinal signaling cells

Typically MSC stands for 'mesenchymal stem cell' and is a specific type of multipotent adult stem cell with the capacity to differentiate into various cell types. These cells can transform into cells that make up our skeletal tissues, such as bone, cartilage, and muscle cells, as well as fat cells [*PMID19023885*]. The multipotent nature of MSCs offers enormous potential for treating a variety of diseases and conditions, ranging from osteoarthritis to autoimmune disorders.

Found in a multitude of tissues throughout the body, mesenchymal stem cells are most commonly sourced from bone marrow, adipose tissue, and umbilical cord tissue. The diversity of their origins adds another layer of versatility to MSCs, making them accessible and adaptable for therapeutic uses. For instance, bone marrow-derived MSCs have shown promise in treating hematological diseases, while adipose-derived MSCs are frequently investigated for their potential in tissue engineering and regenerative medicine.

One of the defining characteristics of MSCs is their unique ability to not only regenerate damaged tissues but also to modulate immune responses. They secrete various cytokines and growth factors that inhibit inflammatory responses and stimulate tissue repair. This immunomodulatory role places MSCs at the forefront of therapies aimed at conditions like multiple sclerosis, Graft-Versus-Host Disease, and other autoimmune disorders where immune system modulation can be therapeutic. This will be discussed in detail in Part III.

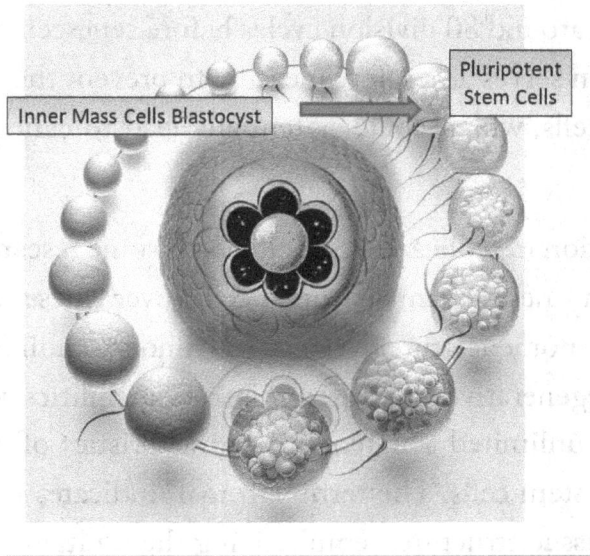

Fig.4: Pluripotent cells originate from the inner mass of the blastocyst and then become more specialized until they are finally adult cells. They have a finite life cycle. In theory, Pluripotent cells can assist in making any tissue. Blastocyst derived 'pluripotent cells' are an early stage of 'stem cells' but they are not toti-potent! The next stage is considered 'mulitpotent MSCs' as they can only differentiate into specialized tissues. [PMID21396235, PMID33371306]

Medicinal Signaling Cell:

Moreover, MSCs have garnered attention for their capacity to secrete bioactive molecules that aid in tissue repair and regeneration. They release a wide array of signaling molecules and growth factors, which can act in an autocrine or paracrine manner to promote tissue recovery. This feature enables them to create a more favorable environment for healing, going beyond merely replacing damaged cells.

However, MSCs are the subject of ongoing debate within the scientific community, primarily due to the semantics surrounding their name. Although termed "stem cells," they have a limited lifespan, undergoing around 80 division cycles before senescence. This natural limitation serves as a safety measure to prevent the uncontrolled growth of cells, which could potentially lead to cancerous formations.

This limitation in replicative capacity leads some researchers to prefer the term "mesenchymal stromal cells" over "mesenchymal stem cells." This nomenclature reflects the understanding that while they have regenerative and differentiative capabilities, they may not possess the unlimited self-renewal characteristics of totipotent or pluripotent stem cells. The term "stromal" indicates their supportive role in tissue structures, emphasizing the multi-functional roles they play beyond differentiation.

Interestingly, for therapeutic applications, the limited lifespan of MSCs could be considered an advantage. Their finite replication cycle reduces the risk of uncontrolled growth and malignant transformation, which makes them a safer choice for cell-based therapies. In many ways, this "built-in safety feature" addresses one of the significant concerns surrounding stem cell therapies—the potential for tumorigenicity.

While some may argue about whether MSCs fully meet the classical definitions of stem cells, what is undebatable is their utility in clinical settings. Their multi-lineage differentiation potential, combined with their immunomodulatory and tissue reparative capabilities, make them an extremely promising tool in the rfapidly evolving field of regenerative medicine.

In summary, MSCs—whether you term them mesenchymal stem cells, stromal or signaling cells—are a remarkable class of cells with vast therapeutic potential. Their unique characteristics, such as tissue regeneration, immune system modulation, and secretion of growth factors, make them highly promising candidates for a wide range of medical applications, from treating degenerative diseases to mitigating the effects of tissue damage and aging.

By focusing on their unique properties and understanding the intricacies of their function, we can open up new avenues for treatments that could revolutionize healthcare in ways we are only beginning to understand.

CD Markers

How MSCs are characterized by Research

Researchers have been using varying methodologies for the isolation, expansion, and characterization of mesenchymal stem cells (MSCs). This diversity in experimental approaches makes it increasingly challenging to make direct comparisons between study results, thereby impeding progress in this important area of research. In an effort to establish some level of standardization, the Mesenchymal and Tissue Stem Cell Committee of the International Society for Cellular Therapy has put forth minimal criteria to define human MSCs. According to these guidelines, first, MSCs must adhere to plastic surfaces under standard culture conditions. Second, they must display specific surface markers, expressing CD105, CD73, and CD90, while lacking expression of CD45, CD34, CD14 or CD11b, CD79α or CD19, and HLA-DR. Third, they should have the ability to differentiate into osteoblasts, adipocytes, and chondroblasts when cultured in vitro. [PMID16923606]

What is a CD marker?

CD markers, also known as clusters of differentiation markers, are specific molecules present on the surface of cells. They serve as identifiers that help to categorize and define cell types, particularly those of the immune system. CD markers are usually glycoproteins, but they can also be lipids or other types of molecules. They are often used in research and medical diagnostics to distinguish between different cell populations based on the presence or absence of these markers.

The "CD" nomenclature is followed by a number, which is essentially a label for that particular marker. For example, CD4 is a marker predominantly found on helper T cells, while CD8 is primarily found on cytotoxic T cells. Both are essential components of the adaptive immune system.

CD markers play various roles in cellular function including, but not limited to, cell signaling, cell adhesion, and immune response modulation. For example, CD40 and CD40L interactions are crucial for B-cell development and activation, and CD28 is an important co-stimulatory molecule for T cells.

In the context of mesenchymal stem cells (MSCs), CD markers like CD105, CD73, and CD90 are often used to define and isolate these cells. The absence of certain markers (Fig. 5), such as CD45, CD34, and others, is equally important for confirming that the cells in question are indeed MSCs and not other cell types like hematopoietic stem cells or other immune cells.

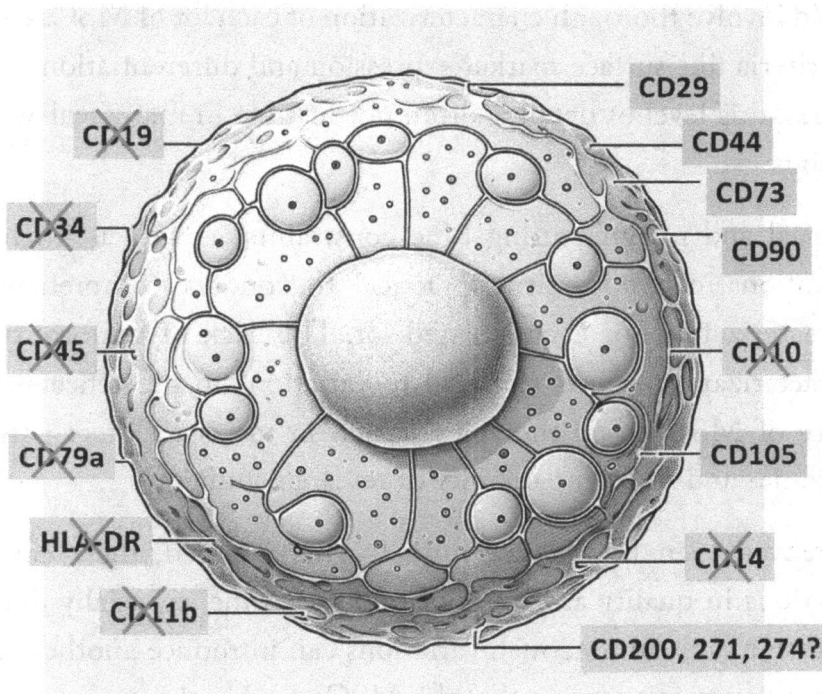

Fig.5: CD markers present and absent in MSCs (compared to fibro-blasts) [PMID16923606, PMID31216380]

The use of CD markers is particularly common in techniques like flow cytometry, which allows for the sorting and analysis of individual cells based on their specific markers. This enables researchers and clinicians to better understand the composition of complex cell mixtures and to isolate particular cell types for further study or therapeutic applications.

Characterizing Natural sources of 'MSCs'

Indeed, the complexity of natural sources for mesenchymal stem cells (MSCs), such as adipose tissue, bone marrow, and umbilical cord tissue, presents challenges in ensuring consistency and quality across different batches of isolated MSCs. While ideal practices would involve thorough characterization of each lot of MSCs based on criteria like surface marker expression and differentiation capabilities, this level of detail is often not feasible in many real-world settings.

Clinical and manufacturing time constraints, as well as financial limitations, can make it impractical to conduct comprehensive characterization for each isolated lot. This lack of uniformity in characterization efforts can lead to variations in the efficacy and safety of MSC-based therapies, which in turn can affect patient outcomes and the comparability of research studies.

Moreover, even if cells are initially characterized, there can be variations in quality and composition over time, especially during expansion and culture. Such variations can introduce another layer of complexity in ensuring that the MSCs used in therapies meet all the expected criteria for efficacy and safety.

These issues underscore the need for standardized protocols and guidelines for MSC isolation, expansion, and characterization. Industry-wide standards could help in achieving more consistent and reliable results, thereby accelerating progress in this promising field of regenerative medicine.

Efforts have been made by regulatory bodies and scientific organizations to set guidelines and minimal criteria for MSC characterization, but implementation often varies due to the reasons mentioned above. As the field advances, it will be increasingly important to find a balance between rigorous scientific characterization and the practical needs of clinical and manufacturing processes.

MSC - Why 'Stem Cell' Is the Wrong Word

The term "stem cell therapy" often conjures images of embryonic stem cells and the ethical debates surrounding their use. However, in current clinical settings, the phrase frequently misrepresents the actual cells being used for treatment. Embryonic stem cells are considered 'totipotent', meaning they have the ability to form an entire organism, including extraembryonic tissues like the placenta. They are sourced from the inner cell mass of a blastocyst (Fig. 4), an early-stage embryo. This is the focal point of much ethical debate, as obtaining these cells often destroys the embryo, raising moral and ethical questions that have yet to be conclusively addressed on a societal level.

Contrastingly, the majority of stem cell therapies today use mesenchymal stem cells or **"medicinal signaling cells"** (MSC) which are adult stem cells typically harvested from bone marrow, adipose tissue, or umbilical cord tissue {PMID26079607}. These cells are not totipotent but are instead considered pluri- or multipotent. They have been shown to differentiate into a limited range of cell types—such as bone, cartilage, and fat cells—related to their tissue of origin. MSCs have a finite life cycle and because these cells are not derived from embryos, they sidestep the ethical issues linked to embryonic stem cell use.

It's essential to emphasize that MSCs are usually harvested from consenting adult donors or are sourced from umbilical cords or other birth tissue that would otherwise be discarded after birth. No embryo or fetal life is harmed. Thus, they do not involve the destruction of a potential life and are generally considered ethically non-controversial. These cells also carry a lower risk of tumor formation compared to embryonic stem cells, which adds another layer of safety in their application.

Furthermore, MSCs are often favored in clinical settings due to their immunomodulatory properties. These cells can modulate immune responses, reducing inflammation [PMID26079607] and aiding in tissue repair. Such characteristics make MSCs particularly promising for treating autoimmune diseases and promoting tissue regeneration, broadening their applicability far beyond what embryonic stem cells can offer.

Another point of distinction comes in the form of immune rejection. Embryonic stem cells, with their extensive differentiation potential, also carry a higher risk of immune system rejection when transplanted into a recipient. MSCs, in contrast, have shown to be more "immune-privileged," meaning they are less likely to be rejected by the host's immune system, although the mechanisms for this are still not entirely understood.

Mesenchymal vs Stromal Cell

Often "MSC" is translated as "Mesenchymal Stromal Cell". Here is why this is not quite correct. "Mesenchymal" and "Stromal" are two terms frequently used in cell biology, particularly in the context of stem cell research. While they are often used interchangeably, they have distinct origins and implications. The term "mesenchymal stromal cells" is sometimes used to describe cells that were initially thought to be stem cells due to their ability to differentiate into various cell types. However, as research progressed, it became evident that not all cells in the mesenchymal population are true stem cells.

This term reflects the understanding that while these cells have regenerative and differentiation capabilities, they may not all possess the classical stem cell properties of self-renewal and multipotency.

Mesenchymal - Origin and Definition:

The term "mesenchymal" originates from embryology and refers to the mesenchyme, an embryonic tissue. The mesenchyme is a type of connective tissue that is derived primarily from the mesoderm, one of the three germ layers in early embryonic development.

Mesenchymal cells are characterized by their ability to migrate and differentiate into a variety of cell types, including osteoblasts (bone cells), chondrocytes (cartilage cells), myocytes (muscle cells), and adipocytes (fat cells).

In the context of stem cell research, mesenchymal stem cells are a specific type of multipotent stem cells that can differentiate into various cell types belonging to the connective tissue lineage.

MSCs are known for their potential in regenerative medicine, owing to their ability to differentiate, their immunomodulatory properties, and their capacity to secrete a range of bioactive molecules.

Stromal - Origin and Definition:

"Stromal" refers to the stroma, which is the supportive framework of a biological tissue. Stromal cells are therefore the cells that make up this supportive framework, providing structural support to the functional cells in a tissue.

In many tissues, stromal cells have roles in the microenvironment, influencing functions such as cell growth, migration, and differentiation.

Stromal Cells in Bone Marrow

In the bone marrow, stromal cells include a variety of cell types such as fibroblasts, endothelial cells, and adipocytes. They provide support and regulate the microenvironment for hematopoietic stem cells (blood-forming stem cells).

Stromal cells, unlike mesenchymal stem cells (MSCs), do not possess 'stemness'. While stromal cells provide structural support and contribute to the microenvironment in tissues, they lack the ability to self-renew and differentiate into multiple cell types, which are key characteristics of stem cells.

To summarize, while "mesenchymal" refers to cells originating from the embryonic mesenchyme with the ability to differentiate into various tissue types, "stromal" pertains more broadly to cells that provide structural and functional support within tissues. In the context of regenerative medicine, these terms often overlap but have nuances that reflect the evolving understanding of cell biology and stem cell research.

More Stem cell terminology

Additionally, the term "stem cell" often implies a level of pluripotency that MSCs do not possess. This misconception can lead to unrealistic expectations about the therapeutic capabilities of MSC-based treatments. Patients might believe that these cells have miraculous healing properties, which could set the stage for disappointment or even exploitation.

While MSCs do have promising regenerative properties, they are not a cure-all. Their effectiveness varies depending on various factors, such as the method of delivery, the health of the recipient, and the specific condition being treated. Therefore, labeling MSC-based treatments as "stem cell therapy" might inadvertently contribute to the hype, rather than accurately portraying the therapy's limitations and capabilities.

In the scientific community, some researchers prefer to use the term "mesenchymal stromal cells" to more accurately reflect the characteristics and limitations of these cells. The word "stromal" denotes their supportive role in tissue, emphasizing their function without overstating their capabilities, as the term "stem cell" might.

In summary, while MSCs do fall under the broad category of stem cells due to their self-renewal and differentiation capabilities, the term "stem cell therapy" can be misleading when applied to treatments that employ MSCs. The distinction is not merely semantic; it carries implications for patient expectations, ethical considerations, and regulatory oversight. Instead MSC can also be translated as 'Mesenchymal Signaling Cells' as will be discussed later. For these reasons, it's important to use terminology that accurately reflects the nature and potential of the cells being used.

Limited Life Cycle

Mesenchymal stem cells (MSCs), like all cells, do have a finite life span in tissue culture, a phenomenon often referred to as replicative senescence. However, the specific number of cell divisions that MSCs can undergo before reaching senescence can vary and is not strictly fixed at a certain number of divisions.

Replicative senescence in MSCs is characterized by a decline in their proliferative ability and a reduction in their differentiation potential. This process is influenced by several factors:

Telomere Shortening: Each time a cell divides, the telomeres at the ends of its chromosomes become slightly shorter. When they reach a critically short length, the cell enters senescence and stops dividing. This is a natural process that acts as a kind of cellular 'clock'. [PMID28454681]

Stress and Culture Conditions: The conditions under which MSCs are cultured can significantly impact their lifespan. Factors such as oxygen concentration, growth factors, and the density of the cells in culture can influence how many times the cells can divide before senescing.

Donor Variability: The source of MSCs can also affect their replicative lifespan. Cells from older donors, for example, may have a shorter lifespan compared to those from younger donors.

Genetic and Epigenetic Factors: Individual genetic differences and epigenetic modifications (changes in gene expression) can also play a role in determining the replicative lifespan of MSCs.

Types of Stem Cell Therapies- Allogeneic, Autologous and Wharton's jelly

Here is a brief list of the types of 'stem cells terminologies' that can be introduced in the context of stem cell therapy and regenerative medicine:

Umbilical Cord Mesenchymal Stem Cells (UC-MSCs):

These are harvested from the Wharton's jelly of the umbilical cord (or other placental or amniotic tissue). They can be used allogeneically, which means they can be donated from one individual to another without the need for a direct genetic match.

Allogeneic Stem Cells:

Stem cells donated from a genetically non-identical member of the same species. Allogeneic stem cell transplants were traditionally commonly used in conditions where the immune system is involved, such as in hematopoietic stem cell transplantation for leukemia. However allogeneic cells usually are considered immunogenic in allopathic medicine. This is not the case in umbilical tissue.

Autologous Bone Marrow Stem Cells (BMSCs):

These are harvested from the individual's own bone marrow. They are used in autologous transplants, where a person's own cells are used to minimize the risk of immune rejection. These procedures have a high occurrence of side effects. According to this large study provided by one of the biggest stem cell therapy companies about 14% of the patients treated from their own bone marrow had serious side effects: A multi-center analysis of adverse events among two thousand, three hundred and seventy two adult patients undergoing adult autologous stem cell therapy for orthopedic conditions. [PMID27026621]

Adipose-Derived Stem Cells (ADSCs or SVFs):

Obtained from adipose tissue (fat), these stem cells sometimes called Adipose stromal vascular fraction (SVF) cells can be used for autologous transplants. They are easier to obtain in large quantities compared to bone marrow stem cells and have been used in cosmetic surgery, wound healing, and other regenerative procedures.

But as in any surgical procedure, even liposuction has a small risk of serious side effects such as embolism.

Once again, the term "stromal vascular fraction" (SVF) might be misleading if interpreted to imply that all cells within this fraction possess stemness. While SVF contains a heterogeneous mixture of cells, including mesenchymal stem cells (MSCs), endothelial cells, pericytes, and immune cells, not all of these cells exhibit stemness (stem cell properties).

Induced Pluripotent Stem Cells (iPS Cells):

These are adult cells that have been genetically reprogrammed to an embryonic stem cell-like state, meaning they can differentiate into almost any cell type. iPSCs hold significant promise for creating patient-specific therapies and are a key area of research for regenerative medicine.

Chimeric Antigen Receptor T-Cells (CAR-T):

Although not stem cells, CAR-T cells are a form of cellular therapy that involves reprogramming a patient's T-cells to target and attack cancer cells. The T-cells are genetically modified to express a chimeric antigen receptor (CAR) specific to the cancer cells' antigens. [PMID38855617]

What does Science say about MSCs

MSC Differentiation Potential

Mesenchymal stem cells (MSCs) do have 'stemness' potential which can be demonstrated in the lab. Here's an overview of the cell types into which MSCs can differentiate:

Cell Types Differentiated from MSCs

Osteoblasts: MSCs can differentiate into osteoblasts, the cells responsible for bone formation. This capability is fundamental to their use in bone repair and regeneration.

Chondrocytes: Chondrocytes are the cells that form cartilage. MSCs can differentiate into chondrocytes, making them valuable in treating cartilage defects and osteoarthritis.

Adipocytes: MSCs can become adipocytes, which are fat cells. This property is explored in research focused on metabolic diseases and tissue reconstruction.

Myocytes: Myocytes are muscle cells, and MSCs have the potential to differentiate into various types of muscle cells, including cardiac muscle cells, though this is a more complex and less efficient differentiation pathway.

Neural Cells: There is evidence that MSCs can differentiate into neural cell types under certain conditions, although this is not their primary lineage. The extent and functional significance of this differentiation are areas of ongoing research.

Other Cell Types:

MSCs have also been reported to differentiate into other cell types, such as endothelial cells (which line blood vessels), under specific experimental conditions. However, these differentiation pathways are less typical and require specific inducing factors. EG. The differentiation of MSCs into liver cells (hepatocytes) is an area of growing interest, particularly for liver disease treatment. However, this is not a typical pathway for MSC differentiation, and the efficiency and functionality of the MSC-derived hepatocytes compared to primary hepatocytes are subjects of ongoing research.

While MSCs are primarily known for their ability to differentiate into cell types related to connective tissues such as bone, cartilage, and fat, research is continually uncovering broader potentials, including the possibility of differentiating into hepatocyte-like cells. However, the efficiency and functionality of MSCs in forming non-connective tissue cell types, such as liver cells, are still being explored and refined in research settings. [PMID31357692]

Clarification on Mesenchymal Stem Cells (MSCs) in Therapeutic Applications

Mesenchymal stem cells (MSCs) indeed possess stemness potential, which is the ability to self-renew and differentiate into multiple cell types. This potential is well-demonstrated in laboratory settings. However, the behavior of MSCs in therapeutic applications, particularly in allogeneic injections or intravenous (IV) therapy, can differ significantly:

- Stemness in the Lab: In controlled laboratory environments, MSCs can be induced to differentiate into various cell types, such as osteoblasts, chondrocytes, and adipocytes. This ability underpins their potential in regenerative medicine.

- Therapeutic Use: When MSCs are used in allogeneic injections or IV therapy, they are less likely to engraft permanently in the recipient's tissues. Instead of implanting and differentiating, their primary therapeutic effects are mediated through paracrine signaling:

- Paracrine Effects: MSCs secrete a range of bioactive molecules, including cytokines, growth factors, and exosomes, which modulate the local environment, reduce inflammation, and promote tissue repair and regeneration.

- Immunomodulation: MSCs have potent immunomodulatory properties, which help in reducing immune responses and inflammation. This makes them useful in treating autoimmune diseases and inflammatory conditions.

In conclusion, While MSCs have demonstrated stemness potential in laboratory settings, their primary mode of action in allogeneic injection or IV therapy is through their paracrine effects rather than direct implantation and differentiation. This understanding is crucial for appreciating the therapeutic benefits and mechanisms of MSCs in clinical applications.

Why choose Umbilical Cord MSCs?

The crucial reason for the use of Umbilical cord derived stem cells (UC-MSC) vs autologous MSCs relates to the 'age' of the cells and the regenerative message they provide. Nature has provided a rich stem cell tissue within the umbilical cord to regenerate the mothers tissue after birth and help grow the fetus. Wharton's jelly is a gelatinous substance that is found in the umbilical cord. It is a type of connective tissue that surrounds the blood vessels in the cord, providing support and protection. Wharton's jelly also prevents compression of the blood vessels in the umbilical cord, which can impede the flow of oxygen and nutrients to the developing fetus and is an ideal tissue for MSC cells. UC-MSCs come with an array of regenerative growth factors and anti-inflammatory cytokines. These go to work right away:

1) Studies show that inflammatory markers such as TNFalpha and IL-6 are reduced by 80% in the first few days. [PMID22008910, PMID6022321, PMID34102486, PMID33363221]

2) Following is the production of fresh exosomes (included by tissue culture production). The exosomes deliver a message to reduce old scar tissue. (see also Part III)

3) MSCs can become implanted and stay in your body for months to stimulate your own body cells to regenerate proper tissue such as cartilage or tendons. [PMID17656645]

In Summary, Wharton's jelly is an excellent source for mesenchymal stem cells (MSCs) because it contains a high concentration of these cells, which have the ability to differentiate into various cell types, such as bone, cartilage, and fat cells.

One of the advantages of using MSCs derived from Wharton's jelly is that they are relatively easy to isolate and expand in the laboratory. Unlike other sources of MSCs, such as bone marrow or adipose tissue, which require invasive procedures to obtain, Wharton's jelly can be obtained non-invasively from the umbilical cord after childbirth.

Additionally, MSCs derived from Wharton's jelly have been shown to have unique properties compared to MSCs from other sources. For example, they have a higher proliferation rate and a greater potential for differentiation, which makes them an attractive option for use in regenerative medicine applications.

Once again, each of these cell types has unique applications and considerations in both research and clinical settings. The field continues to evolve rapidly as new discoveries enhance our understanding of the capabilities and potential uses of various stem cell types. It is beyond the scope of this book to decide which therapy is the best approach for an individual situation. Powerful MSCs with minimal side effects can be derived from your own adipose tissue. However, these SVF cells lack the same regenerative properties as umbilical cord tissue-derived MSCs (UC-MSCs). SVF cells often have lower viable cell counts and require an invasive procedure for extraction. In contrast, UC-MSCs and their regenerative "message," as you will see later on, provide an easier and faster treatment option with fewer side effects compared to deriving cells from your own body.

Graft-Versus-Host Disease

Much confusion exists on this topic within allopathic medicine, necessitating clarification. The primary reason for the limited use of umbilical cord tissue is the mistaken belief in a potential "transplant reaction." This misconception is deeply ingrained in Western thinking, despite a lack of scientific or clinical evidence to support it. Graft-Versus-Host Disease (GVHD) is a major concern in the context of cell transplantation, especially when cells are sourced from another donor (allogeneic transplantation). Ironically, MSC therapy is often employed to alleviate the symptoms of GVHD

[PMID29947972]. Here is how GVHD relates to the different types of stem cells mentioned:

Umbilical Cord Mesenchymal Stem Cells (UC-MSCs):

UC-MSCs are considered to have low immunogenicity, which means they are less likely to provoke an immune response in the recipient. This characteristic potentially reduces the risk of GVHD when UC-MSCs are used in allogeneic transplants.

Allogeneic Stem Cells:

In allogeneic transplants, stem cells from a donor are transplanted to a recipient. This can lead to GVHD if the immune cells from the donor recognize the recipient's tissues as foreign and mount an immune response against them.

Autologous Bone Marrow Stem Cells (BMSCs):

Since autologous transplants involve the patient's own cells, there is no risk of GVHD. This is one of the key advantages of using autologous BMSCs While autologous bone marrow (BM) transplants eliminate the risk of Graft-Versus-Host Disease (GVHD), they can still have serious side effects due to several factors:

- Conditioning Regimen: Before the transplant, patients undergo high-dose chemotherapy and/or radiation therapy to destroy their existing bone marrow. This conditioning regimen can cause significant side effects, including infections, bleeding, and organ damage due to the toxicity of the treatment.

- Engraftment Syndrome: During the engraftment phase, when the new bone marrow starts to produce blood cells, patients can experience a range of symptoms, including fever, rash, and fluid retention, which can sometimes be severe.

- Infection Risk: The immune system is weakened during the period when the new bone marrow is not yet fully functional, making patients highly susceptible to infections.

- Organ Damage: The chemotherapy or radiation used in the conditioning regimen can cause long-term damage to organs such as the heart, liver, and kidneys.

- Recurrent Disease: There is always a risk that the underlying disease, such as cancer, could recur even after an autologous transplant.

- Graft Failure: Although rare, there is a possibility that the transplanted bone marrow may not engraft properly, leading to a failure to produce new blood cells.

These factors contribute to the complexity and potential severity of side effects associated with autologous bone marrow transplants, despite the absence of GVHD.

Adipose-Derived Stem Cells (ADSCs):

Like autologous BMSCs, ADSCs used in an autologous manner do not carry a risk of GVHD because the cells originate from the patient's own body.

Induced Pluripotent Stem Cells (iPS Cells):

iPSCs can be derived from the patient's OWN cells, thus eliminating the risk of GVHD when used in an autologous context. However, if iPSCs are used allogeneically, the risk of GVHD would still exist. Therefore these iPSC therapies are not without side effects. Despite their promise, one of the **significant** challenges that remain is understanding and mitigating immune rejection, even when iPSCs are derived from a patient's own cells.

Chimeric Antigen Receptor T-Cells (CAR-T):

CAR-T cell therapy is designed to be autologous, with the patient's own T-cells being engineered to attack their cancer cells, which means GVHD is not a concern. However, if CAR-T cells were to be developed from allogeneic sources, there could be a risk of GVHD and Therefore these therapies can have significant side effects.

GVHD remains one of the significant challenges in artificial stem cell transplantation, especially with allogeneic transplants from tissue culture derived sources. Researchers continue to explore methods to mitigate this risk, including the use of immunosuppressive drugs, T-cell depletion techniques, and the application of tolerance-inducing strategies.

However this generally excludes Mesenchymal stem cells (MSCs), due to their immunomodulatory properties. On the contrary, they are being studied for their potential to prevent or treat GVHD.

In general, Graft-Versus-Host Disease (GVHD) is most commonly associated with transplants involving immune cells, which is a particular concern in hematopoietic stem cell transplantation (HSCT) rather than solid organ transplantation. In HSCT, the transplanted stem cells can give rise to immune cells that may attack the recipient's body tissues, leading to GVHD. Here are some more examples in detail:

Hematopoietic Stem Cell Transplantation:

In HSCT, which is a common treatment for conditions like leukemia and lymphoma, the patient receives hematopoietic stem cells from a donor. These stem cells will develop into new blood cells, including immune cells, in the recipient's body. If these new immune cells recognize the recipient's body as foreign, they may attack, leading to GVHD.

Immune Response:

GVHD occurs when donor T-cells, a type of white blood cell, become activated and proliferate in response to the recipient's tissues. The disease can manifest in acute or chronic forms and can affect multiple organs, including the skin, liver, gastrointestinal tract, and lungs.

Organ Transplantation:

In the context of organ transplantation, such as kidney or liver transplants, the concern is more about organ rejection rather than GVHD. This happens when the recipient's immune system attacks the transplanted organ. While GVHD is not a concern in solid organ transplantation, it is theoretically possible if donor immune cells within the transplanted organ become active against the recipient's tissues, but this is rare and not the primary concern as it is with HSCT.

iPSCs and CAR-T Cells:

Induced pluripotent stem cells (iPSCs) and chimeric antigen receptor T-cells (CAR-T) therapies are typically autologous, which means they are derived from the patient's *own* cells, so they do not carry a risk of GVHD. However, research is ongoing into the allogeneic use of these cells, which would require careful management to avoid GVHD.

In summary, Mesenchymal Stem Cells (MSCs) are different from most other allogeneic transplants:

The risk of GVHD with MSCs, including those derived from umbilical cord tissue, is much lower because MSCs have in fact immunomodulatory properties that may actually help suppress the immune response and prevent GVHD. This is one of the reasons why there is interest in using MSCs to treat or prevent GVHD. The unique immunomodulatory properties of MSCs provide a potential avenue for reducing the risk of GVHD, and their use in this context is still an area of active research. This will be discussed in detail in chapter 3. [PMID15494428]

MSCs have special CD markers

As discussed above, Mesenchymal stem cells (MSCs) are known for their immunomodulatory properties, which include the ability to modulate the immune response and potentially reduce the incidence or severity of Graft-Versus-Host Disease (GVHD). This function is partially attributed to the expression of specific surface molecules, known as CD markers. The interaction of these markers with the immune system plays a key role in the immunomodulatory effects of MSCs.

Here are some key CD markers and related molecules that are significant in the context of MSCs and their immunomodulatory functions [PMID24578244, PMID25797907]:

CD73, CD90, and CD105: These are the standard markers used to identify MSCs. While they are primarily used for identification and confirmation of MSCs, they also play roles in cell adhesion and signaling. Their presence is part of the criteria established by the International Society for Cellular Therapy (ISCT) for defining MSCs.

HLA-G: Human Leukocyte Antigen G (HLA-G) is an immunomodulatory molecule that MSCs can express. HLA-G contributes to the immunosuppressive effects of MSCs and plays a role in preventing the rejection of the transplanted cells by the recipient's immune system.

PD-L1 (CD274): Programmed Death-Ligand 1 (PD-L1) is a molecule that MSCs can express, which helps in suppressing T-cell activity. This expression is a mechanism by which MSCs can modulate immune responses and potentially reduce GVHD.

CD200: MSCs express CD200, a molecule involved in the regulation of immune responses. The interaction of CD200 with its receptor, CD200R, found on immune cells, can lead to the suppression of immune responses. [PMID32849489]

Indoleamine 2,3-Dioxygenase (IDO): While not a CD marker, IDO is an enzyme expressed by MSCs that can suppress immune responses by depleting tryptophan, an amino acid necessary for T-cell proliferation.

In addition, CD271 has been described as the most specific marker for the characterization and purification of human bone marrow mesenchymal stem cells. This marker has been shown to be specifically expressed by these cells.

It's important to note that the immunomodulatory effects of MSCs are not solely dependent on these markers but involve a complex interplay of various soluble factors, cell-to-cell contact, and other mechanisms. MSCs can modulate the immune system through both cell-contact dependent mechanisms and the secretion of soluble factors, leading to an altered immune environment that can suppress inappropriate immune responses, such as those seen in GVHD.

Furthermore, the expression of these markers and molecules can be influenced by the conditions in which MSCs are cultured and by the local environment in the recipient's body. Research continues to explore how these factors can be optimized to enhance the therapeutic potential of MSCs, particularly in the context of preventing or treating

CD Marker	MSCs	Fibroblasts
CD34	Absent	Absent
CD45	Absent	Absent
CD73	Present	Present
CD90	Present	Present
CD105	Present	Absent/Variable
CD14	Absent	Absent
CD19	Absent	Absent
CD79a	Absent	Absent
HLA-DR	Absent	Absent
CD29	Present	Present
CD44	Present	Present
CD166	Present	Absent/Variable
CD10	Absent	Absent

Table 1a: Common markers present and absent in MSCs vs. fibroblasts

Common Markers: Both MSCs and fibroblasts share some surface markers, such as CD73, CD90, and CD44. This overlap can sometimes complicate the distinction between these cell types.

Unique Markers: CD105 and CD166 are typically present in MSCs but are less commonly expressed in fibroblasts. The presence of these markers can help differentiate MSCs from fibroblasts.

Absence of Hematopoietic Markers: Both cell types lack hematopoietic markers such as CD34 and CD45, which helps to distinguish them from hematopoietic stem cells.

Immune Markers: Both MSCs and fibroblasts are typically negative for immune cell markers like CD14, CD19, CD79a, and HLA-DR. Common Markers: Both MSCs and fibroblasts share some surface markers, such as CD73, CD90, and CD44. This overlap can sometimes complicate the distinction between these cell types.

Unique Markers: CD105 and CD166 are typically present in MSCs but are less commonly expressed in fibroblasts. The presence of these markers can help differentiate MSCs from fibroblasts. Absence of Hematopoietic Markers: Both cell types lack hematopoietic markers such as CD34 and CD45, which helps to distinguish them from hematopoietic stem cells. Immune Markers: Both MSCs and fibroblasts are typically negative for immune cell markers like CD14, CD19, CD79a, and HLA-DR. [PMID36997513]

iPSC - CD Markers

As mentioned above, Induced pluripotent stem cells (iPSCs), discovered by Dr. Shinya Yamanaka, have opened new frontiers in regenerative medicine and personalized therapy. Despite their promise, one of the significant challenges that remain is understanding and mitigating immune rejection, even when iPSCs are derived from a patient's own cells. Additionally, specific CD markers play a critical role in identifying and characterizing iPSCs and their differentiated progeny.

iPSCs and Immune Rejection

Autologous iPSCs: iPSCs that are derived from a patient's own cells, theoretically minimizing the risk of immune rejection because they are genetically identical to the donor.

Immune Response: Despite this genetic similarity, some studies have shown that autologous iPSCs can still elicit an immune response. This response may be due to mutations acquired during the reprogramming process or the expression of antigens not present in the original somatic cells.

Allogeneic iPSCs: iPSCs that are derived from a donor and used in another individual show immune challenges. These cells are more likely to provoke an immune response because of genetic differences between the donor and recipient, similar to traditional organ transplants.

Mitigation Strategies:

Immunosuppressive Therapy: Use of drugs to suppress the immune system and prevent rejection, although this comes with potential side effects. These are similar to organ transplants causing GVHD as discussed above.

Gene Editing: Techniques like CRISPR can be used to modify iPSCs to reduce their immunogenicity, either by knocking out specific antigens or introducing genes that promote immune tolerance.

Immune Evasion: Engineering iPSCs to express molecules that help them evade the immune system, such as PD-L1, which can inhibit T-cell activity.

CD Markers in iPSCs

iPSCs, which are pluripotent, express a unique set of CD markers that distinguish them from other stem cell types, including MSCs. [PMID23378912, PMID29686294, PMID38093391]

Pluripotency Markers:

- SSEA-4 (Stage-Specific Embryonic Antigen-4): Expressed on the surface of pluripotent stem cells, including iPSCs.

- TRA-1-60 and TRA-1-81: Surface antigens used to identify pluripotent stem cells.

- CD90 (Thy-1): Another marker associated with stemness, although not exclusively.

Distinct CD Markers of iPSCs and MSCs

Induced pluripotent stem cells (iPSCs) and mesenchymal stem cells (MSCs) are both powerful tools in regenerative medicine, but they exhibit distinct characteristics, including their surface markers, known as CD (cluster of differentiation) markers. These markers are used to identify and differentiate between various cell types and their states of differentiation.

Comparison of CD Markers:

Here's a comparison (Table 1b) to highlight the distinct CD markers between iPSCs and MSCs. As you can see, these genetically altered cells have little resemblance to MSCs. The distinct CD markers expressed by iPSCs and MSCs reflect their different biological roles and states of differentiation. iPSCs, characterized by markers such as SSEA-4, TRA-1-60, and key pluripotency transcription factors like Oct4, Sox2, and Nanog, are capable of differentiating into any cell type in the body. In contrast, MSCs, identified by markers such as CD73, CD90, and CD105, are multipotent stem cells with a more limited differentiation potential, primarily into mesodermal lineages. Understanding these differences is crucial for researchers and clinicians in selecting the appropriate cell type for specific therapeutic applications.

CD Marker	iPSCs	MSCs
SSEA-3	Present	Absent
SSEA-4	Present	Absent
TRA-1-60	Present	Absent
TRA-1-81	Present	Absent
Oct4	Present	Absent
Sox2	Present	Absent
Nanog	Present	Absent
CD73	Absent	Present
CD90	Absent	Present
CD105	Absent	Present
CD44	Absent	Present
CD29	Absent	Present
CD34	Absent	Absent
CD45	Absent	Absent

Table 1b: Common markers present and absent in iPSC vs. MSC

In summary, iPSCs hold immense potential for personalized and regenerative medicine, but challenges such as immune rejection need to be addressed. Understanding the role of CD markers in identifying and characterizing iPSCs and their derivatives is crucial for advancing their clinical application. Strategies to mitigate immune rejection, including immunosuppressive therapy, gene editing, and engineering immune evasion, are key areas of ongoing research. By overcoming these challenges, iPSC technology can move closer to its full therapeutic potential

Modern 'stem cell' therapy

Exosomes, Secretome extracts and other MSC derived products

As we venture further into the realm of modern stem cell therapy, it's crucial to broaden our perspective beyond the cells themselves and explore the innovative products derived from these cells. Recent advancements have spotlighted the role of exosomes, secretome extracts, and other mesenchymal stem cell (MSC)-derived products, which are proving to be just as pivotal as the stem cells from which they originate.

The Emergence of Exosomes:

Exosomes are tiny vesicles secreted by cells, including MSCs. They play a vital role in cell communication by transporting proteins, lipids, and RNA to other cells. In the context of stem cell therapy, exosomes derived from MSCs have garnered attention due to their ability to replicate many of the regenerative effects of the stem cells themselves. They are seen as a promising therapeutic tool because they lack the complexity and risks associated with cell transplantation.

The Secret to Secretomes

The 'message' of MSCs or other stem cells are called 'secretomes' and may be the solution to many clinical applications. The secretome refers to the collection of factors secreted by cells, which includes growth factors, cytokines, and other signaling molecules. The 'MSC-Secretome', in particular, is rich in bioactive molecules that can modulate inflammation [PMID26079607], promote tissue repair, and enhance healing. Unlike direct stem cell therapies, using the secretome can provide a cell-free approach to treatment, reducing risks associated with stem cell transplantation such as immune rejection or tumor formation.

MSC-Derived Products:

In addition to exosomes and secretomes, other products derived from MSCs, such as conditioned media (the solution in which MSCs have been cultured), are being explored for their therapeutic potential. These products contain a blend of bioactive molecules that can contribute to tissue regeneration and healing.

Clinical Applications:

The clinical applications of these MSC-derived products are diverse, ranging from wound healing and skin rejuvenation to the treatment of degenerative diseases and immune modulation. Their versatility and lower risk profile make them attractive alternatives or adjuncts to traditional stem cell therapies. The field of MSC-derived products is rich with ongoing research and development. Scientists are continually discovering new ways these products can be used, understanding their mechanisms of action, and optimizing their therapeutic potential.

Regulatory and Ethical Considerations:

With the introduction of these novel therapies come regulatory challenges and ethical considerations. Ensuring the safety, efficacy, and quality of these products is paramount. Regulatory agencies are evolving their frameworks to accommodate these new therapies, ensuring they meet stringent standards before being approved for clinical use.

The advent of novel therapies using exosomes, secretomes, and other mesenchymal stem cell (MSC)-derived products is reshaping the landscape of regenerative medicine. These advancements bring unique regulatory challenges and ethical considerations, distinct from those associated with traditional live cell therapies.

Regulatory Perspective on Cell-free Products:

A significant advantage of using exosome and secretome-based therapies lies in their classification as cell-free products. Since these therapies do not involve live cells, they bypass some of the primary concerns associated with cell-based therapies, such as issues of immune rejection and the complexities of cell viability during storage and transportation.

Simplified Ethical Landscape:

Unlike therapies that use embryonic stem cells or even certain allogeneic adult stem cells, exosome and secretome therapies do not delve into ethically complex territories. There's no risk of immune rejection typically associated with allogeneic cell transplants, and they avoid the ethical debates surrounding the use of embryonic cells.

Safety and Efficacy:

While these therapies may have a simpler ethical and regulatory path, ensuring their safety and efficacy remains paramount. Regulatory agencies are tasked with evaluating these products to ensure they are safe, effective, and produced using standardized, quality-controlled processes.

Regulatory Evolution: As the field of regenerative medicine continues to evolve, so too must the regulatory frameworks governing it. This involves developing specific guidelines and protocols for the production, testing, and application of exosome and secretome therapies.

Clinical Trials and Research:

Comprehensive clinical trials and research are essential to establish the therapeutic potential and safety profile of these novel treatments. Continued research is necessary to fully understand their mechanisms of action and long-term effects.

Informed Consent and Patient Education: With novel therapies, it is crucial to have clear and transparent patient education and consent processes. Patients should be fully informed about the nature of the therapy, its potential benefits, and risks.

Future Implications:

As we navigate the complexities of introducing these new therapies into clinical practice, we must also consider their long-term implications on healthcare. This includes understanding how they may alter treatment paradigms and the potential impact on healthcare costs and accessibility.

In this book, we will explore the intricacies of these advanced therapies derived from MSCs. We will look into how they are changing the face of treatment in various medical fields, offering innovative solutions without the complexities of live cell therapies. As you continue reading, you'll gain insights into how these therapies are developed, regulated, and applied, providing a comprehensive view of this cutting-edge area of medicine.

We will also explore the exciting advancements in MSC-derived products such as exosomes and secretomes. We'll delve into how they are revolutionizing the field of regenerative medicine, offering new pathways to healing and recovery that were once thought impossible. As you journey through these pages, you will gain an appreciation for the intricacies of these therapies and the immense potential they hold for the future of medicine.

Part II

A Brief History of Stem Cell Discovery

Landmarks and Pioneers

Pinpointing the "first" instance of a specific type of medical treatment, such as the injection of allogeneic umbilical cord mesenchymal stem cells (UC-MSCs) into a human, can be challenging due to the complexities of medical research history and the numerous concurrent studies in various parts of the world. Clinical trials and experimental therapies often progress in parallel, and records of "firsts" might not always be meticulously documented or may be subject to debate.

That said, the use of umbilical cord-derived MSCs for therapeutic purposes has been explored for decades but especially since the early 2000s. One of the early milestones in the field was the discovery and characterization of MSCs in umbilical cord tissue. Following these discoveries, researchers began investigating the potential therapeutic applications of these cells.

One of the earlier documented uses of UC-MSCs in a clinical setting was in the treatment of Graft-Versus-Host Disease (GVHD) and other conditions where the immunomodulatory properties of MSCs could be beneficial. However, identifying a singular "first" instance of such a treatment being administered is not straightforward, as clinical trials and experimental treatments are often conducted simultaneously around the globe.

The study by S. Knudtzon in 1974 would have been groundbreaking at the time as it demonstrated the presence of progenitor cells in human cord blood capable of forming granulocytic colonies in vitro. Knudtzon, S. (1974): "In vitro growth of granulocytic colonies from circulating cells in human cord blood" [PMID4811820]

This research laid the groundwork for using umbilical cord blood as a source of hematopoietic stem cells for transplantation, which is a standard practice today for treating various blood and immune system diseases. The isolation and growth of these progenitor cells would have shown that cord blood, like bone marrow, contains cells capable of giving rise to different types of blood cells, thus opening up new avenues for research and therapeutic applications. The article already demonstrated in 1974 the ability of colony formation from cord blood cells derived from 3 adult mothers.

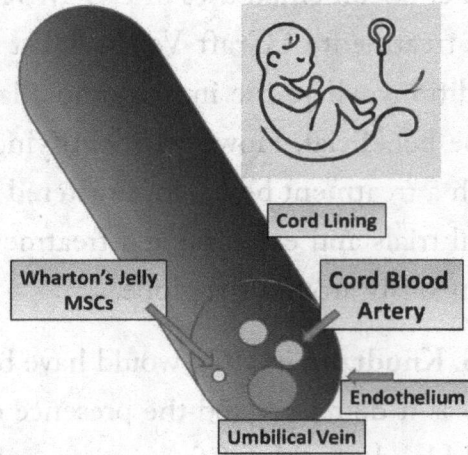

Fig. 6: Schematic of Wharton's jelly (WJ) from umbilical cord tissue. MSCs can be derived from various compartments.

Dr. Arnold I. Caplan: A Pioneer in Stem Cell Research

One man stands out in the history of early Stem cell discovery: Dr. Arnold I. Caplan, a renowned ure in the field of stem cell research, has made substantial contributions that have significantly shaped our understanding of regenerative medicine (with over 390 pubmed citations). Often referred to as the "father of the mesenchymal stem cell (MSC)," Dr. Caplan's work has been pivotal in identifying and characterizing these cells, which have become a cornerstone of stem cell therapy and tissue engineering.

Discovery and Naming of MSCs:

One of Dr. Caplan's most notable achievements is his work in the early 1990s that led to the identification and characterization of MSCs. He was instrumental in coining the term "mesenchymal stem cells." His research demonstrated that these cells, derived from bone marrow, have the capacity to differentiate into various cell types, including bone, cartilage, and fat cells.

Pioneering Regenerative Medicine:

Dr. Caplan's work has been foundational in the field of regenerative medicine. He proposed and developed the concept that MSCs could be used therapeutically, not only for their potential to differentiate into various tissue types but also for their remarkable ability to modulate immune responses and aid in tissue repair.

Advancing Tissue Engineering:

Beyond stem cell biology, Dr. Caplan has significantly contributed to the field of tissue engineering. His research has provided insights into how MSCs can be used in conjunction with biomaterials to create tissue constructs for repairing or replacing damaged tissues.

Educational and Advisory Roles:

A distinguished educator and thought leader, Dr. Caplan has served as a mentor to numerous students and researchers in the field. His advisory roles have extended to various scientific boards and committees, helping to shape policies and guide research in stem cell science and regenerative medicine.

Public Advocacy for Stem Cell Research:

Dr. Caplan has been a vocal advocate for ethical and responsible stem cell research. He has consistently emphasized the importance of rigorous scientific methodology and ethical considerations in the exploration and application of stem cell therapies. His advocacy extends to public education, where he has worked to demystify the science behind stem cells and address the misconceptions surrounding the field.

Prolific Research and Publications:

With hundreds of publications to his name, Dr. Caplan's research has been widely cited and has significantly influenced the direction of stem cell research. His work continues to inspire new investigations and applications in the field, bridging the gap between basic science and therapeutic innovations.

Legacy and Impact

Dr. Arnold I. Caplan's groundbreaking work has not only advanced our fundamental understanding of MSCs but also opened new avenues for treating a wide array of diseases and injuries. His vision and dedication have placed him at the forefront of regenerative medicine, making him a true pioneer whose impact will be felt for generations to come in the fields of stem cell research and tissue engineering. His legacy is evident in the growing number of MSC-based therapies and the continued exploration of the vast potential these cells hold.

In summary, the discovery and characterization of mesenchymal stem cells (MSCs) have been pivotal milestones in the field of regenerative medicine and there certainly are many research groups and facilities that contributed. Here are some more key references that mark significant moments in the early research and understanding of MSCs:

Friedenstein, A. J., Chailakhyan, R. K., & Gerasimov, U. V. (1987). Bone marrow osteogenic stem cells: in vitro cultivation and transplantation in diffusion chambers. Cell and Tissue Kinetics, 20(3),

263-272. [PMID 3690622] This is one of the foundational studies by Alexander Friedenstein and colleagues, who were among the first to describe the osteogenic potential of bone marrow cells, a landmark in the discovery of MSCs.

Caplan, A. I. (1991). Mesenchymal stem cells. Journal of Orthopaedic Research, 9(5), 641-650. Arnold Caplan, who is often credited with coining the term "mesenchymal stem cell," discusses the multipotent nature of these cells in this influential paper. [PMID 1870029]

Pittenger, M. F., Mackay, A. M., Beck, S. C., Jaiswal, R. K., Douglas, R., Mosca, J. D., ... & Marshak, D. R. (1999). Multilineage potential of adult human mesenchymal stem cells. Science, 284(5411), 143-147. This seminal paper by Pittenger and colleagues provides evidence of the multipotent nature of MSCs, demonstrating their ability to differentiate into osteoblasts, adipocytes, and chondroblasts. [PMID10102814]

Prockop, D. J. (1997). Marrow stromal cells as stem cells for nonhematopoietic tissues. Science, 276(5309), 71-74. Darwin Prockop's work contributes significantly to the understanding of the potential of marrow stromal cells (another term for MSCs) in regenerating nonhematopoietic tissues. [PMID9082988]

Le Blanc, K., Tammik, L., Sundberg, B., Haynesworth, S. E., & Ringdén, O. (2008). Mesenchymal stem cells for treatment of steroid-resistant, severe, acute Graft-Versus-Host Disease: a phase II study. Lancet, 361(9374), 1579-1586. This study demonstrates the clinical application of MSCs, particularly in treating severe conditions like Graft-Versus-Host Disease. [PMID18468541]

Zuk, P. A., Zhu, M., Mizuno, H., Huang, J., Futrell, J. W., Katz, A. J., ... & Hedrick, M. H. (2001). Multilineage cells from human adipose tissue: implications for cell-based therapies. Tissue engineering, 7(2), 211-228. Patricia Zuk and colleagues' research on isolating multipotent stem cells from human adipose tissue broadened the understanding of MSC sources. [PMID11304456]

Here is a most recent review by Caplan: "Mesenchymal stem cell perspective: cell biology to clinical progress. MSCs were isolated and described about 30 years ago and now there are over 55,000 publications on MSCs readily available. Here, we have focused on human MSCs whenever possible." [PMID31815001]

These references provide just a glimpse into the early stages of MSC peer reviewed research published in some of the most renown journals. The field has significantly evolved since these initial discoveries, and newer research continues to expand our understanding of MSCs, their characteristics, and their therapeutic potential.

Early Publications

Studies and Findings

The use of amniotic fluid, amniotic membrane, and placental tissue in medical treatments, particularly for burn wound care, has a long history. In addition, placental tissue was used in Chinese Medicine for centuries. These biological materials are known for their healing properties, which include anti-inflammatory effects, the promotion of epithelialization, and the reduction of scar tissue formation. Below are some key historical points and studies related to their use:

Early Use in Burn Treatment since 1910:

Amniotic Membranes have been used in clinical practice for over a century. Mainly, it was used in surgery as a biological coating. Ingraldi 2023 [PMID37888195] summarizes: "Fetal membranes were first used in the 1900s to successfully treat acute and chronic traumatic wounds, burns, ulcers, and as a novel skin substitute for grafting [PMID17862406, PMID15416059]. The amniotic membrane's inherent elasticity allows it to conform to complex contoured surfaces, which led to its application in many reconstructive procedures, including the creation of artificial vaginas, and treating chronic complex wounds in diabetic patients" [PMID12683248, PMID22592624].

The use of amniotic membrane for burn treatment dates back to the early 20th century. In 1910, Davis was one of the first to report the use of amniotic membranes for skin transplantation in burn wounds. Davis, JW. states in 1910: **"The use of human amniotic allograft (HAA) in various surgical procedures, has been proven to facilitate bone growth and both soft tissue and cartilage healing".** Skin transplantation with a review of 550 cases at the Johns Hopkins Hospital. Johns Hopkins Med J. 1910;15:307–96; [PMID17862406]; **Stern, M. 1913: "The grafting of preserved amniotic membrane to burned and ulcerated surfaces, substituting skin grafts"** [JAMA. 1913;60(13):973-974.]

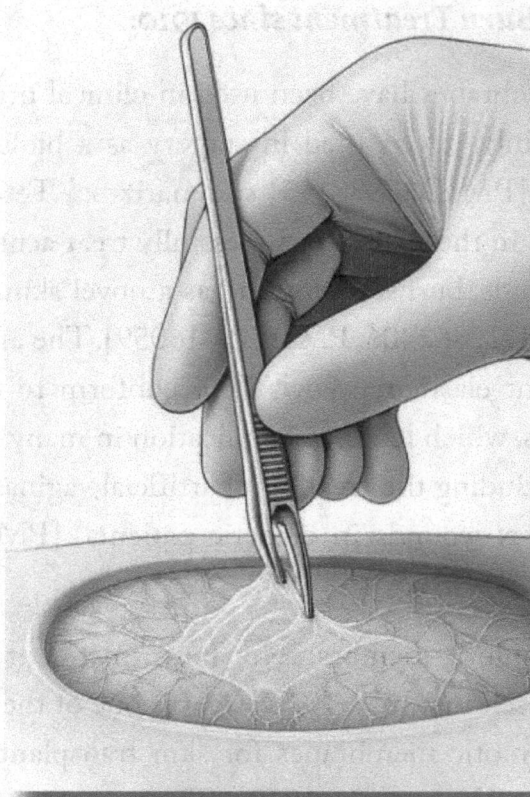

Fig.7: Schematic use of amniotic membranes in skin grafts of burns and wounds **as early as 1910**

Pioneering Studies:

As mentioned above Stern, M. (1913) and Troensegaard-Hansen, E. (1950) reported the use of amniotic membrane as a biological dressing for burn wounds, which aided in pain relief and facilitated healing. [PMID15416059]

Amniotic Fluid and Wound Healing:

Research has indicated that amniotic fluid contains various growth factors and cytokines that are essential for fetal growth and development, and these components can promote wound healing when applied to burn injuries.

Placental Tissue in Regenerative Medicine:

The placental tissue has been used not only for wound dressing but also in regenerative medicine due to its rich content of stem cells and growth factors.

Modern Applications:

With advancements in cell biology Revisiting the Role of Amniotic Membrane Dressing in Acute Large Traumatic Wounds: A Randomized Feasibility Study at a Level 1 Trauma Centre - [PMID38025497] and the establishment of cell banks, amniotic and placental tissues have been processed into various forms, such as grafts and patches, for clinical use. Using Amniotic Membrane as a Novel Method to Reduce Post-burn Hypertrophic Scar Formation: A Prospective Follow-up Study - [PMID28529415]

Regulatory Considerations:

The use of these tissues is subject to regulatory oversight to ensure safety and efficacy, with agencies like the FDA providing guidance for their use in therapeutics. Unfortunately, in over 110 years of clinical studies and hundreds of research publications, this important discovery was never really implemented in the standard treatment of burns.

In summary Kesting 2008 [PMID18849850] concludes: "Randomized clinical trials favored the use of amnion in burns in the first place for promotion of wound healing and in the second place for its comfortable and less dressing changes. Antimicrobial effects, pain relief, reduction of fluid, and scar formation were demonstrated additionally." Role of Allogenic Amniotic Membrane in Burn Treatment | Journal of Burn Care & Research | Oxford Academic (oup.com)

Chinese Medicine and Placental Tissue Use - Historical Practices and Modern Implications

Of course thousands of years ago Chinese Doctors did not have labs and tissue culture possibilities. Instead they had a preparation method to preserve placental tissue for its medicinal use.

Traditional Chinese Medicine (TCM) has a rich history of using placental tissue, known as "ZiHeChe," for various health benefits. Placental tissue is considered a powerful source of Qi (vital energy) and blood in TCM, and its use dates back centuries. Below is an elaboration on the historical practices and the modern implications of growth factors and other tissue regenerative factors found in placental tissue.

Chinese Historical Practices - ZiHeChe (Placenta) in TCM:

In TCM, the human placenta has been used as an ingredient in various formulations. It is classified as a tonic and is traditionally believed to replenish Qi, nourish the blood, promote general vitality, and support kidney essence.

Medicinal Preparations:

The placenta would be dried and ground into a powder before being used in different medicinal preparations. It has been used to treat conditions such as fatigue, infertility, impotence, and insufficient lactation.

Philosophical Basis: The philosophy of TCM posits that the placenta contains life-giving and sustaining properties as it is the source of nourishment for the developing fetus. Thus, it is believed to have profound rejuvenating effects when consumed.

Historical Texts: Ancient Chinese medical texts, such as "Bencao Gangmu" (Compendium of Materia Medica), describe the placenta's use and are still referenced today in the practice of TCM.

Modern Implications - Bioactive Components:

Scientific investigations into placental tissue have identified a range of bioactive components, including growth factors like epidermal growth factor (EGF), fibroblast growth factor (FGF), and placental growth factor (PlGF). These factors can stimulate cell growth and proliferation, which is crucial for tissue repair and regeneration.

Regenerative Medicine: In modern regenerative medicine, these growth factors are being studied for their potential in promoting the healing of wounds, the regeneration of tissues, and the treatment of degenerative diseases.

Cosmetics and Pharmaceuticals: Extracts from placental tissue are now used in the cosmetic industry for their supposed anti-aging and skin-rejuvenating properties. Additionally, pharmaceutical companies are exploring placental extracts for their therapeutic potential.

Scientific Validation: While TCM has long asserted the benefits of placental tissue, modern science seeks to validate these claims through rigorous testing and clinical trials to understand the mechanisms by which these growth factors work and to ensure their safety and efficacy.

Ethical Considerations:

With the advent of these modern applications, there is a parallel increase in ethical considerations, particularly concerning the source and consent for the use of human placental tissues.

In conclusion, the use of placental tissue in Traditional Chinese Medicine serves as an early example of regenerative therapy that has extended into modern medical practices. The growth factors and other regenerative components found in placental tissue continue to be of significant interest in both scientific research and applied therapeutics, bridging ancient practices with contemporary biomedical advancements.

As a side note, the use of human placental tissues in medical and cosmetic products has been met with various ethical, legal, and safety concerns. As a result, the use of animal placental tissue, most commonly from sheep, has become an alternative.

Sheep placenta is rich in nutrients and growth factors and is considered to have beneficial properties similar to those of human placenta. Here are some points regarding the modern use of sheep placenta:

Bioactive Components: Sheep placenta contains numerous growth factors, hormones, and other bioactive molecules that are believed to contribute to its regenerative and healing properties.

Cosmetic Industry: In the cosmetic industry, sheep placenta extracts are often found in skin creams and serums. They are marketed as anti-aging products that can help rejuvenate the skin, improve its elasticity, and reduce wrinkles.

Nutritional Supplements: Some health supplements are made from sheep placenta and are marketed as natural remedies that promote general well-being, vitality, and anti-aging benefits.

Regenerative Medicine: There is growing interest in the potential use of ovine placenta-derived cells and extracts in regenerative medicine, due to their regenerative properties and the lower risk of zoonotic disease transmission compared to other animals.

Safety and Ethical Concerns: While sheep placenta is considered a safer and more ethical alternative to human placental tissue, it is still subject to safety and ethical regulations to ensure that products are free from diseases and that animals are treated humanely.

Regulatory Oversight: Regulatory bodies in various countries oversee the use of animal tissues in consumer products, ensuring that they are processed in a way that mitigates the risk of disease transmission and adheres to safety standards.

Research and Clinical Trials: Studies and clinical trials are ongoing to better understand the efficacy and potential therapeutic applications of sheep placenta in medicine.

Cultural Acceptance: The acceptance of sheep placenta in health and cosmetic products varies globally, depending on cultural attitudes towards the use of animal products in consumer goods.

Sustainability: The use of sheep placenta also raises questions about sustainability and environmental impact, which are increasingly important considerations for consumers and manufacturers.

Alternative Sources: In response to both demand and concerns, research continues into alternative sources of bioactive molecules that can mimic the beneficial properties of placental tissue without using animal or human tissues.

In summary, while the use of human placental tissues in products is restricted, sheep placenta has become a popular alternative, especially in the cosmetic and supplement industries. The purported benefits drive its use, although the industry is regulated to ensure consumer safety and ethical standards are met.

Discovery of Wharton's Jelly and Tissue Culture

Research and Applications - Discovery of Wharton's Jelly

Wharton's jelly is a gelatinous substance found within the umbilical cord. It was first described in the 17th century by Thomas Wharton, an English anatomist. Wharton's jelly surrounds and protects the umbilical vessels, which connect the developing fetus to the placenta.

Anatomical and Physiological Significance: This substance is rich in a type of sugar-protein complex called glycosaminoglycans, particularly hyaluronic acid, which gives it a jelly-like consistency. This unique composition provides the cord with resilience and flexibility, protecting the vital blood vessels against compression.

Source of Mesenchymal Stem Cells (MSCs):

In the late 20th and early 21st centuries, researchers discovered that Wharton's jelly is not just a structural material but also a rich source of MSCs. These cells are less mature than other adult stem cells, such as those from bone marrow, and have a higher expansion potential, making them highly promising for therapeutic applications.

The Development of Tissue Culture: A Milestone in Research

The advent of tissue culture represents a pivotal moment in the history of biological and medical research. This technique, which involves the growth and maintenance of cells or tissues outside their natural environment in a controlled setting, has revolutionized our understanding of cellular processes and opened up new avenues for scientific exploration.

Significance of Tissue Culture in Research- In Vitro Study of Cells:

Tissue culture has enabled scientists to study cells in isolation, providing a clearer understanding of their biology, physiology, and genetics. This has been instrumental in unraveling the complexities of cellular functions and interactions.

Drug Discovery and Development: The ability to grow cells and tissues in vitro has been crucial for the pharmaceutical industry. It allows for the screening of potential drug candidates, toxicity testing, and the development of new therapeutics.

Cancer Research: Tissue culture has been particularly valuable in cancer research, enabling the study of tumor cells and their responses to various treatments. It has facilitated the development of targeted therapies and personalized medicine approaches.

Regenerative Medicine: The technique has laid the foundation for regenerative medicine, including tissue engineering and stem cell therapy. By growing cells and tissues in the lab, scientists can create grafts for transplantation and explore new treatments for a range of diseases.

Vaccine Production: Tissue culture is also essential for the production of vaccines. It allows for the cultivation of viruses and the development of attenuated or inactivated vaccines, contributing significantly to public health.

Model Systems for Research: Cultured cells and tissues serve as model systems for studying disease mechanisms, testing hypotheses, and exploring the effects of various environmental factors on cellular behavior.

Historical Perspective

The development of tissue culture can be traced back to the early 20th century, with pioneers like Ross Harrison and Alexis Carrel making significant contributions to the establishment of the technique. Since then, advancements in culture media, growth conditions, and imaging technologies have continually enhanced the capabilities of tissue culture.

In conclusion, the development of tissue culture has been a cornerstone in the advancement of biological and medical research. It has provided scientists with powerful tools to dissect the intricacies of cellular life, develop life-saving therapies, and push the boundaries of our understanding of the living world. As technology continues to evolve, the potential of tissue culture in research and medicine will undoubtedly expand, promising new discoveries and innovations in the years to come.

Technical Development of Tissue Culture:

The practice of tissue culture involves growing cells in an artificial environment, typically a gel-like substrate in a petri dish or flask. This technique was developed and refined during the 20th century and has become essential for studying cell behavior, drug development, and regenerative medicine.

Tool for Research and Medicine: Tissue culture allows for the examination of cells in a controlled environment, where researchers can study the effects of drugs, toxins, and various physiological conditions without experimenting on living organisms.

Regenerative Medicine Applications: In the context of regenerative medicine, tissue culture techniques are crucial for expanding and manipulating stem cells, including those from Wharton's jelly, to sufficient quantities for therapeutic use.

Advancements in Tissue Engineering: Tissue culture has also facilitated advancements in tissue engineering, where researchers create complex tissues and even organoids that mimic organs, which can be used for transplantation or to model diseases in the lab.

Ethical and Accessible Source of Stem Cells: Cells from Wharton's jelly provide an ethically non-controversial and readily accessible source of stem cells. Unlike embryonic stem cells, their use does not involve the destruction of embryos, and unlike bone marrow stem cells, their collection is non-invasive. UC-MSCs can easily be studied in tissue cultures.

Isolation Techniques of Umbilical MSCs

Growing umbilical cord-derived mesenchymal stem cells (MSCs) in tissue culture involves a series of steps to ensure their proliferation and maintenance in vitro. Here's a general overview of the process:

- Collection: The umbilical cord is collected after birth with proper consent and following ethical guidelines.

- Processing: The cord is then cleaned and dissected to isolate the Wharton's jelly or cord blood, which is rich in MSCs.

- Enzymatic Digestion: The tissue is subjected to enzymatic digestion, typically using collagenase, to release the MSCs.

- Centrifugation and Seeding: The cell suspension is centrifuged to obtain a pellet, which is then resuspended in culture medium and seeded into culture flasks.

- Culture Medium: A suitable culture medium, such as Dulbecco's Modified Eagle Medium (DMEM) supplemented with fetal bovine serum (FBS), antibiotics, and growth factors, is used to support cell growth.

- Incubation: The cells are incubated at 37°C in a humidified atmosphere with 5% CO_2.

- Passaging: Once the cells reach confluence (typically 70-80%), they are detached using trypsin-EDTA and passaged to new flasks to maintain optimal growth conditions.

Characterization and Expansion

Characterization: The isolated MSCs are characterized by their morphology (fibroblast-like shape), adherence to plastic, and expression of specific surface markers (e.g., CD73, CD90, CD105) while lacking hematopoietic markers (e.g., CD34, CD45).

Expansion: The MSCs can be further expanded in culture to obtain the desired number of cells. This expansion process needs to be carefully monitored to maintain the cells' undifferentiated state and functional properties.

Cryopreservation

Freezing: For long-term storage, MSCs can be cryopreserved in a freezing medium containing a cryoprotectant like dimethyl sulfoxide (DMSO) and stored in liquid nitrogen.

Thawing: When needed, the cells can be rapidly thawed and cultured again for further use or experimentation.

Applications of MSC tissue cultures: Cultured umbilical MSCs are used in various research and clinical applications, including regenerative medicine, tissue engineering, and studying cell biology and disease mechanisms.

Tissue culture of mesenchymal stem cells (MSCs) and the production of exosomes in vitro are important areas of research in regenerative medicine and cell therapy. Here's an overview of how MSCs are cultured and how exosomes are produced and harvested in a laboratory setting:

Tissue Culture of MSCs and Exosome production

Isolation of MSCs: MSCs can be isolated from various sources, including bone marrow, adipose tissue, and umbilical cord tissue. The tissue is processed to obtain a cell suspension, which is then plated in culture flasks.

Expansion in Culture: MSCs are cultured in a suitable growth medium, typically containing fetal bovine serum (FBS), essential nutrients, and growth factors. The cells are maintained at 37°C in a humidified atmosphere with 5% CO_2.

The culture medium is regularly changed to remove waste products and replenish nutrients. MSCs are passaged when they reach a certain confluence to prevent overgrowth and maintain their undifferentiated state.

Characterization of MSCs: Cultured MSCs are characterized by their fibroblast-like morphology, adherence to plastic, and expression of specific surface markers such as CD73, CD90, and CD105. They should also lack hematopoietic markers like CD34 and CD45.

Exosome Production and Harvesting

Specifically, the production of the 'MSC message', namely 'exosome-vesicles' is of interest here. This process however is highly dependent on the source of MSCs and how the cells are treated in tissue cultures. Some exosomes are harvested directly from birth tissue without propagation in tissue culture.

Exosome Secretion: MSCs naturally secrete exosomes as part of their intercellular communication. These exosomes carry proteins, lipids, and nucleic acids that can influence the behavior of recipient cells.

Collection of Conditioned Medium: To harvest exosomes, the conditioned medium (the medium in which MSCs have been cultured) is collected. This medium contains the exosomes secreted by the MSCs.

Exosome Isolation: Various methods can be used to isolate exosomes from the conditioned medium, including ultracentrifugation, size exclusion chromatography, and immunoaffinity capture. Ultracentrifugation is one of the most common methods, where the medium is centrifuged at high speeds to pellet the exosomes.

Purification and Characterization: The isolated exosomes are further purified and characterized by their size, morphology, and marker expression. Common exosomal markers include CD9, CD63, and CD81. Techniques like nanoparticle tracking analysis (NTA), transmission electron microscopy (TEM), and Western blotting are used for characterization.

Storage: Purified exosomes can be stored at -80°C for long-term use. Proper storage is crucial to maintain their integrity and biological activity. However exosome products are also exceptionally stable at ambient temperatures.

Exosome Contents

Mesenchymal stem cell (MSC) exosomes contain proteins as well as other biomolecules. The protein content of MSC exosomes can include a variety of functional and structural proteins. Here are some key points about the protein content in MSC exosomes:

- Surface Proteins: MSC exosomes contain surface proteins, including tetraspanins (e.g., CD9, CD63, CD81), integrins, and adhesion molecules, which are important for exosome targeting and uptake by recipient cells.

- Cytosolic Proteins: The interior of MSC exosomes contains cytosolic proteins, including enzymes, heat shock proteins, and signaling molecules that can influence various cellular processes in recipient cells.

- Growth Factors and Cytokines: MSC exosomes can carry growth factors and cytokines that play a role in tissue repair, immune modulation, and anti-inflammatory responses. Examples include TGF-ß, VEGF, and IL-10.

- Extracellular Matrix Proteins: Some exosomes contain extracellular matrix proteins, such as fibronectin and laminin, which can contribute to tissue remodeling and repair.

- Proteins Involved in Exosome Biogenesis: Proteins involved in the formation and release of exosomes, such as ALIX and TSG101, are also present in MSC exosomes.

Therapeutic Proteins: Due to their content, MSC exosomes are being studied and clinically used for their potential therapeutic applications in regenerative medicine, immunomodulation, and as delivery vehicles for therapeutic proteins and other molecules. [PMID22619510, PMID29807782]

Proteomic Analysis of MSC Exosomes: Research studies have used proteomic techniques to identify and characterize the protein content of MSC exosomes. These studies have revealed a wide array of proteins that are involved in various biological functions. Overall, the protein content of MSC exosomes is diverse and plays a crucial role in their biological functions and therapeutic potential. [PMID34884740]

Stability

The stability of proteins can be enhanced when they are packaged in exosomes. Exosomes provide a protective environment that can shield encapsulated proteins from various degradative processes. Here are some reasons why protein stability is enhanced when packaged in exosomes:

- Protection from Degradation: Exosomes encapsulate proteins within a lipid bilayer, protecting them from proteolytic enzymes and other degradative factors present in the extracellular environment. [PMID28255367]

- Stable Microenvironment: The interior of exosomes provides a stable microenvironment that can preserve the structure and functionality of proteins. This can be particularly important for sensitive proteins that might otherwise degrade or denature in the extracellular space. [PMID21640565]

- Extended Circulation Time: Exosomes can circulate in the bloodstream for extended periods, allowing for more efficient delivery of their protein cargo to target cells. This prolonged circulation time can enhance the stability and bioavailability of the encapsulated proteins.

- Targeted Delivery: The surface proteins and lipids on exosomes facilitate their targeted delivery to specific cells or tissues, reducing the likelihood of non-specific degradation.

- Reduced Immune Clearance: Exosomes are generally less immunogenic than other delivery systems, which can reduce their clearance by the immune system and enhance the stability of their protein cargo. [PMID36726968]

Applications for Exosomes

MSC-derived exosomes are being explored for their therapeutic potential in regenerative medicine, drug delivery, and as biomarkers for disease diagnosis and monitoring.

The tissue culture of MSCs and the production of exosomes are critical processes in the study of cell-based therapies and regenerative medicine. Understanding how to efficiently culture MSCs and harvest their exosomes opens up new avenues for research and potential therapeutic applications.

In conclusion, growing umbilical cord-derived MSCs in tissue culture requires careful attention to isolation, culture conditions, and characterization to ensure the cells retain their stemness and functional properties. These cultured cells hold great promise for advancing our understanding of stem cell biology and developing novel therapeutic approaches.

The discovery of Wharton's jelly as a valuable source of MSCs and the advancement of tissue culture techniques have both greatly enriched the toolkit available to researchers and clinicians. They offer a synergistic platform where the potential of regenerative therapies can be explored, refined, and brought to clinical reality, providing hope for the treatment of a myriad of diseases and injuries.

Artificial stem cells and The Collapse of Embryonic Stem Cell Research

The use of fetal and embryonic stem cells in research and therapy has been a subject of ethical controversy for many decades. While these cells have significant potential for regenerative medicine due to their pluripotency and ability to differentiate into any cell type, their use raises complex moral and ethical issues.

Ethical Controversies Around Fetal Stem Cells

Source of Fetal Cells:

Fetal stem cells are typically derived from aborted fetuses or from fetal tissue that results from elective abortions. This raises ethical concerns regarding the respect for potential human life and the consent process involved in donating fetal tissue for research.

Alternatives: The availability of alternative sources of stem cells, such as adult stem cells and induced pluripotent stem cells (iPSCs), which do not involve the destruction of potential human life, has led to ethical debates on whether the use of fetal stem cells is justifiable.

Consent and Exploitation: Ethical considerations also extend to the consent process for obtaining fetal tissue and the potential for exploitation of vulnerable populations in the procurement of such tissue.

The Fall of Embryonic Stem Cell Research

Moral Concerns: Embryonic stem cell research involves the destruction of human embryos, which many consider to be morally unacceptable. This has led to significant opposition and calls for restrictions on such research.

Legal and Funding Restrictions: Due to ethical concerns, many countries have implemented strict regulations on embryonic stem cell research. In some cases, this has included restrictions on funding, which has hindered the progress of research in this area.

Shift to Alternative Sources: The ethical controversies surrounding embryonic stem cells have contributed to a shift in focus towards alternative sources of pluripotent stem cells, such as iPSCs. iPSCs can be generated from adult cells and do not involve the destruction of embryos, making them ethically less contentious.

Public Perception and Trust: The ethical debates around embryonic stem cell research have also impacted public perception and trust in stem cell research as a whole. Addressing these ethical issues is crucial for maintaining public support and advancing the field responsibly.

The ethical controversies surrounding fetal and embryonic stem cells have had an unfortunate and significant impact on the direction of stem cell research. While these cells offer immense potential for understanding human development and treating diseases, ethical considerations have led to a shift towards alternative sources of pluripotent stem cells. Navigating these ethical issues remains a critical challenge in the field of regenerative medicine, requiring a careful balance between scientific progress and respect for ethical principles.

The Discovery of iPSC cells

In 2012, Dr. Shinya Yamanaka was awarded the Nobel Prize in Physiology or Medicine, an accolade he shared with Sir John B. Gurdon. This prestigious award recognized their groundbreaking contributions to the field of stem cell research, which have fundamentally transformed our understanding of cellular development and regeneration.

Dr. Yamanaka's most notable achievement was the discovery of induced pluripotent stem cells (iPSCs). In 2006, he and his team at Kyoto University demonstrated that it is possible to reprogram mature, differentiated cells back into a pluripotent state. This means that adult cells could be reverted to an embryonic-like state, where they have the potential to differentiate into any cell type in the body.

Reprogramming Factors: Yamanaka identified four key transcription factors—Oct4, Sox2, Klf4, and c-Myc—known collectively as the Yamanaka factors. By introducing these factors into adult cells, he was able to induce pluripotency, thus creating iPSCs.

Significance of iPSCs:

Ethical Advantages: iPSCs bypass the ethical issues associated with embryonic stem cells, as they do not require the destruction of embryos.

Disease Modeling: iPSCs can be used to create patient-specific cell lines, which are invaluable for studying disease mechanisms and testing potential treatments in a controlled environment.

Regenerative Medicine: The ability to generate patient-specific pluripotent cells opens up new possibilities for personalized regenerative therapies, reducing the risk of immune rejection.

Impact on Science and Medicine

The discovery of iPSCs has had a profound impact on both basic science and clinical research:

Expanded Research Horizons: Enabled researchers to study the development and differentiation of various cell types from a single source.

Facilitated Drug Development: Allowed for the creation of disease-specific cell models that can be used to screen for new drugs and therapies.

Advanced Personalized Medicine: Provided a pathway for developing personalized treatments that are tailored to the genetic makeup of individual patients.

Dr. Shinya Yamanaka's Nobel Prize-winning work has revolutionized the field of stem cell research. His discovery of iPSCs has not only deepened our understanding of cellular biology but also paved the way for significant advancements in regenerative medicine, disease modeling, and personalized therapy. The implications of his research continue to inspire and drive scientific innovation, offering hope for new treatments and cures for a wide range of diseases.

However as discussed further on in the context of CD markers, iPSC cells have significant immune rejection when used in a non-autologous context. Despite this genetic similarity, some studies have shown that autologous iPSCs can still elicit an immune response. This response may be due to **mutations** acquired during the reprogramming process or the expression of antigens not present in the original somatic cells.

iPSC vs CAR-T vs NK-cells

The generation of 'iPS' and other genetically engineered cells are a topic beyond the scope of this book. For the sake of completeness they need to be mentioned here. Here's a brief comparison of the tissue culture technologies for induced pluripotent stem cells (iPSCs), chimeric antigen receptor T-cell (CAR-T) therapy, and natural killer (NK) cells:

Induced Pluripotent Stem Cells (iPSCs) in Regenerative Medicine

Induced pluripotent stem cells (iPSCs) have become a focal point in regenerative medicine research, particularly in Western countries. Their ability to be derived from a patient's own somatic cells and reprogrammed into a pluripotent state makes them an attractive option for personalized therapies. However, while iPSCs offer significant potential for regenerating tissues and treating various diseases, there are still challenges and side effects that need to be addressed.

Advantages of iPS-cells

Autologous Source: iPSCs can be generated from a patient's own cells, reducing the risk of immune rejection when transplanted back into the same patient.

Pluripotency: Like embryonic stem cells, iPSCs can differentiate into almost any cell type in the body, offering broad therapeutic potential.

Ethical Considerations: iPSCs bypass the ethical concerns associated with the use of embryonic stem cells, as they do not involve the destruction of embryos.

Challenges and Side Effects

Genetic and Epigenetic Abnormalities: Reprogramming somatic cells into iPSCs can introduce genetic mutations and epigenetic changes that may affect the safety and functionality of the derived cells.

Tumorigenicity: One of the major concerns with iPSCs is their potential to form tumors. The reprogramming process can activate oncogenes or fail to completely differentiate the cells, leading to the formation of teratomas or other types of tumors.

Incomplete Differentiation: Achieving complete and controlled differentiation of iPSCs into the desired cell type, such as pancreatic islet cells, remains a challenge. Incomplete or incorrect differentiation can lead to suboptimal function or unwanted side effects.

iPSCs and Pancreatic Islet Cells

The use of iPSCs to generate pancreatic islet cells for the treatment of diabetes is a promising area of research. [PMID33948571] However, ensuring that the iPSC-derived islet cells function correctly and do not elicit adverse effects is crucial. Researchers are working on refining differentiation protocols and developing strategies to minimize the risks associated with iPSC-based therapies.

While iPSCs represent a promising avenue for regenerative medicine, their application, particularly in complex tissues like pancreatic islet cells, requires careful consideration of the potential risks and side effects. Ongoing research aims to address these challenges, improving the safety and efficacy of iPSC-based therapies for a wide range of medical conditions

Reprogramming procedure:

iPSCs are generated by reprogramming adult somatic cells, such as skin or blood cells, into a pluripotent state. This is typically achieved by introducing specific transcription factors (e.g., OCT4, SOX2, KLF4, c-MYC) into the cells using viral vectors, non-viral methods, or small molecules.

Culture Conditions: Once reprogrammed, iPSCs are cultured in specialized media that support their pluripotent state. This includes the use of feeder layers or feeder-free systems with defined media containing growth factors like FGF2.

Differentiation: iPSCs can be differentiated into various cell types by modifying culture conditions and adding specific growth factors or small molecules to direct their fate.

CAR-T Cell Production Technology

Often confused with stem cells. Chimeric Antigen Receptor T-cell (CAR-T) therapy is a new approach in cancer treatment that leverages the body's immune system to target and eliminate cancer cells. It has shown remarkable success in treating certain types of blood cancers, particularly B-cell malignancies like acute lymphoblastic leukemia (ALL) and diffuse large B-cell lymphoma (DLBCL).

How CAR-T Therapy Works

Isolation of T Cells: The process begins with collecting T cells from the patient's blood through a process called leukapheresis.

Genetic Modification: The isolated T cells are then genetically modified in the laboratory to express a chimeric antigen receptor (CAR) on their surface. This CAR is designed to recognize a specific antigen present on the cancer cells.

Expansion: The CAR-T cells are then cultured and expanded in the laboratory to generate millions of these modified cells.

Infusion: Once a sufficient number of CAR-T cells are produced, they are infused back into the patient's bloodstream. Once in the body, the CAR-T cells multiply and seek out the cancer cells expressing the target antigen.

Cancer Cell Destruction: In theory the CAR-T cells bind to the target antigen on the cancer cells and initiate a potent immune response that leads to the destruction of the cancer cells.

Successes and Challenges in CAR-T

Success in Hematologic Cancers: CAR-T therapy has shown remarkable success in treating certain hematologic cancers, leading to long-term remissions in patients who had previously exhausted all other treatment options.

FDA Approvals: Several CAR-T cell therapies have received FDA approval for the treatment of specific blood cancers, including tisagenlecleucel (Kymriah) and axicabtagene ciloleucel (Yescarta).

Challenges and Side Effects: Despite its successes, CAR-T therapy can have serious side effects, including cytokine release syndrome (CRS) and neurotoxicity. These side effects require careful management and monitoring.

Research and Expansion: Ongoing research aims to expand the use of CAR-T therapy to solid tumors, improve its safety profile, and make it more accessible and cost-effective.

CAR-T therapy is sold as an advancement in cancer treatment, offering new hope to patients with certain types of blood cancers. The therapy is also currently expensive and complex, limiting its accessibility to many patients. As research progresses, the hope is that CAR-T therapy will become safer, more effective, and available to a broader range of patients, including those with solid tumors.

However, the body of long term studies is still outstanding to support this technology.

Isolation and Activation procedure:

T cells are isolated from a patient's blood and activated using antibodies that target CD3 and CD28, along with cytokines like interleukin-2 (IL-2) to promote their proliferation.

Genetic Modification: The activated T cells are then genetically modified to express a chimeric antigen receptor (CAR) that recognizes a specific antigen on cancer cells. This is typically done using viral vectors or non-viral methods like electroporation.

Expansion: The CAR-T cells are expanded in culture using media supplemented with cytokines to obtain a sufficient number for therapeutic use.

Infusion: The expanded CAR-T cells are infused back into the patient, where the hope is, they target and destroy cancer cells.

NK Cell Culture Technology: A Key Player in Immunotherapy

Natural Killer (NK) cells are a vital component of the innate immune system, playing a crucial role in the body's first line of defense against infections and tumors. Unlike T cells, which require antigen presentation to become activated, NK cells can recognize and destroy stressed, infected, or cancerous cells without prior sensitization. This unique ability makes them a promising tool in the field of immunotherapy, particularly in the fight against cancer.

Cytotoxic Activity: NK cells are known for their potent cytotoxic activity. They can induce apoptosis (programmed cell death) in target cells through the release of perforin (pore formation in cell membranes) and granzymes or by engaging death receptors.

Recognition Mechanisms: NK cells can distinguish between healthy and abnormal cells through a balance of activating and inhibitory receptors. This balance ensures that NK cells target only cells that display signs of stress, infection, or malignancy.

Cytokine Production: Upon activation, NK cells produce a variety of cytokines, such as interferon-gamma (IFN-γ) and tumor necrosis factor-alpha (TNF-α), which enhance the immune response and help recruit other immune cells to the site of infection or tumor.

Therapeutic Potential of NK Cells

Cancer Immunotherapy: NK cells are being explored as a form of cancer immunotherapy. Their ability to target and kill tumor cells without the need for prior sensitization makes them attractive candidates for adoptive cell transfer therapies.

Infectious Diseases: NK cells play a significant role in the defense against viral infections. Harnessing their antiviral properties is a potential strategy for treating or preventing infectious diseases.

Engineering NK Cells: Similar to CAR-T cell therapy, NK cells can be genetically modified to enhance their specificity and efficacy against cancer cells. Chimeric antigen receptor (CAR)-NK cells are an emerging area of research in this field.

Allogeneic Transplantation: Unlike T cells, NK cells have a lower risk of causing Graft-Versus-Host Disease (GVHD) in allogeneic transplant settings. This makes them a safer option for cell-based therapies involving donor cells.

Clinical Application of NK cells:

Natural Killer cells represent a powerful tool in the arsenal of immunotherapy, with their innate ability to target and eliminate abnormal cells. As research progresses, the therapeutic potential of NK cells continues to expand, offering new hope for the treatment of cancer and infectious diseases. Their unique properties and the ongoing development of NK cell-based therapies highlight the importance of these cells in advancing the field of medicine.

- Isolation: NK cells can be isolated from peripheral blood, umbilical cord blood, or generated from iPSCs or other progenitor cells.

- Activation and Expansion: NK cells are activated and expanded in culture using cytokines such as IL-2, IL-15, or IL-21. Feeder cells or artificial antigen-presenting cells (aAPCs) may also be used to stimulate their growth.

- Genetic Modification (Optional): Similar to CAR-T cells, NK cells can be genetically modified to enhance their specificity and efficacy against cancer cells.

- Infusion: Expanded NK cells can be infused into patients for cancer immunotherapy or as part of adoptive cell transfer protocols.

In summary, each of these tissue culture technologies serves a unique purpose in regenerative medicine and immunotherapy. iPSC production technology focuses on generating pluripotent cells that can differentiate into various cell types for tissue repair and disease modeling. CAR-T cell production is centered on engineering T cells for targeted cancer therapy. NK cell culture technology involves the expansion and activation of NK cells for natural or enhanced cancer immunotherapy. To clarify, the choice of these technologies are not natural but "artificial" or under genetic manipulation! They usually have little in common with MSC therapies. However a combination of these therapies with natural MSCs in the future may be a viable option.

So what do MSC-cells actually do?

The topic of what MSCs actually do, will be discussed in detail in the following chapters, however it is worth discussing again what Dr. Caplan had to say about this topic: As mentioned above, Dr. Arnold I. Caplan, a prominent ure in the field of regenerative medicine, has made significant contributions to our understanding of mesenchymal stem cells (MSCs). One of his key assertions is that MSCs primarily function as "medicinal signaling cells" rather than traditional stem cells. Here's a summary of his perspective on what MSCs are actually doing in the body:

Medicinal Signaling Cells -Immunomodulation:

Dr. Caplan emphasizes the role of MSCs in modulating the immune response. MSCs can secrete various factors that suppress inflammatory responses and promote tissue repair. This immunomodulatory function is crucial in both normal physiology and in response to injury or disease.

Trophic Support:

MSCs provide trophic support to surrounding tissues by secreting growth factors, cytokines, and other molecules. These secreted factors can stimulate tissue repair, support cell survival, and enhance the function of resident cells.

Homing and Recruitment:

MSCs have the ability to home to sites of injury or inflammation, where they can exert their therapeutic effects. Once at the site, MSCs can recruit other cells, including resident stem cells, to participate in the repair and regeneration process. [PMID29190645]

Extracellular Matrix Remodeling:

MSCs contribute to the remodeling of the extracellular matrix (ECM), which is essential for tissue repair and maintaining structural integrity.

Angiogenesis:

MSCs can promote the formation of new blood vessels (angiogenesis), which is important for supplying nutrients and oxygen to damaged tissues and facilitating the removal of waste products.

A Shift in Perspective

Dr. Caplan's view represents a shift from the traditional concept of MSCs as stem cells with a primary focus on differentiation into various cell types. Instead, he highlights the paracrine and regulatory functions of MSCs as being central to their therapeutic potential.

This perspective has implications for the development of MSC-based therapies, suggesting that the therapeutic benefits of MSCs may be derived more from their secreted factors and immunomodulatory effects than from their ability to differentiate and replace damaged cells.

In conclusion, Dr. Arnold I. Caplan's insights into the role of MSCs as medicinal signaling cells have significantly influenced the field of regenerative medicine. By emphasizing the immunomodulatory and trophic functions of MSCs, his work has expanded our understanding of how these cells contribute to tissue repair and homeostasis, paving the way for novel therapeutic approaches using these safe and easily obtainable regenerative cells.

Part III

Scientific Background

Stem Cell Science - Biology and Mechanisms

Understanding the mechanisms of action of drugs and therapies within the complexities of human biology is an ongoing challenge. This is particularly true in the rapidly evolving field of stem cell therapy, where new discoveries frequently adjust our understanding of how these cells operate and interact within the body. Here's a simplified explanation of how stem cells, particularly mesenchymal stem cells (MSCs), are thought to work in therapeutic contexts:

Basic Principles of Stem Cell Function

The basic principles of stem cell science will be discussed below in the light of past and current research and clinical evidence. Keep in mind that the aim of this book is to provide an overview of current clinical applications. A detailed analysis of each clinical condition as well as advanced research studies is far beyond the intention here.

In practice, we can assume the order and importance of each of these mechanisms now but as research takes its course this may change.

Differentiation:

What it means: In theory Stem cells have the capacity to differentiate into various types of cells. This means they can develop into specialized cells (such as bone, cartilage, muscle, or nerve cells) that are needed to repair or replace damaged tissue. However as you will see, this does not seem to be the case in adult stem cell therapy.

Application: In therapies, this property is exploited to regenerate damaged tissues, such as repairing cartilage in osteoarthritis or healing wounds.

Immunomodulation

What it means: Stem cells can modulate the immune system, meaning they can alter immune responses by either enhancing or suppressing them.

Application: This is particularly valuable in treating autoimmune diseases (like rheumatoid arthritis), reducing inflammation, and preventing the rejection of transplanted tissues.

Paracrine Signaling:

What it means: Stem cells secrete factors that act on nearby cells (a process known as paracrine signaling) to promote tissue repair and regeneration. These factors can stimulate local cells to proliferate, prevent cell death, and attract more reparative cells to the site of injury.

Application: This mechanism is crucial in almost all applications of stem cell therapy, from heart regeneration after myocardial infarction to recovery from spinal cord injuries.

Anti-inflammatory Effects:

What it means: Stem cells can release anti-inflammatory molecules that help calm chronic inflammation, which is a common underlying factor in many diseases. [PMID26079607]

Application: This property is beneficial in managing chronic inflammatory diseases, including certain types of heart disease and neurodegenerative conditions.

The Focus on Adult Stem Cells in Regenerative Medicine

In the dynamic field of regenerative medicine, the source of stem cells used in research and therapy is a topic of significant importance and ethical consideration. Here we specifically focus on non-embryonic sources of stem cells. In essence, the use of embryonic or fetal cells over the last decades, which are often mired in controversy and ethical debates, was mainly a topic of experimental research. Here, our emphasis is on the clinical and practical and less controversial applications of adult stem cells in contemporary Regenerative Medicine. In other words, modern clinical regenerative medicine has no connection to the use of embryonic cells. As will be explained below, the term 'stem cell' in itself is not 'proper' anymore, when it comes to modern clinical applications.

In theory, early embryonic stem cells derived from the blastocyst are 'omnipotent' but there are many levels of pluripotent and multipotent 'stem cells' once tissue differentiation is initiated. In contrast,

MSCs are typically considered a late stage of pluripotent fibroblasts. In other words, they have already progressed 'down the road' and become limited in what tissue they can initiate differentiation.

Here are some important points to consider when talking about regenerative medicine:

Distinction in Stem Cell Sources:

It is crucial to differentiate between embryonic, fetal, and adult stem cells in research studies. Each type has unique properties, ethical considerations, and practical applications. This book primarily discusses adult stem cells, such as mesenchymal stem cells (MSCs), and their therapeutic potential.

Embryonic and Fetal Stem Cells:

Embryonic stem cells are derived from the early stages of a fertilized egg and are considered totipotent, meaning they have the potential to develop into any cell type in the body, including entire tissues and organs. Fetal stem cells, which are slightly more differentiated, are obtained from fetal tissues.

As mentioned above already, the use of these cells has been a subject of ethical controversy due to concerns about the moral status of embryos and fetuses.

Therefore the research on fetal cells has been largely terminated in favor of artificial iPS cells and natural MSCs.

The Shift in Regenerative Medicine:

In recent years, there has been a significant shift in the field of regenerative medicine towards using adult stem cells. These cells, obtained from tissues like bone marrow, adipose tissue, and umbilical cord blood, are not surrounded by the same ethical issues as embryonic and fetal stem cells.

Practicality and Efficacy: Adult stem cells, especially MSCs, have proven to be both practical and effective for a wide range of applications. They offer significant regenerative potential without the ethical and practical challenges associated with embryonic stem cells.

Current Focus: The current focus in regenerative medicine is on harnessing the potential of these adult stem cells for therapeutic applications, such as in the treatment of osteoarthritis, heart disease, and other degenerative joint conditions.

A considerable focus exists on the treatment of inflammatory conditions such as autoimmune disease and Polycystic ovary syndrome (PCOS) and infertility.

Future of Regenerative Medicine:

As we continue to explore the possibilities of adult stem cells, the field is moving towards more targeted and personalized therapies. The advancements in this area are likely to redefine therapeutic approaches in many medical fields such as diabetes [PMID33995278]or heart disease. [PMID28387893]

Another focus of stem cell research is on the so-called reverse engineered iPS or Induced pluripotent stem cells. These are genetically altered fibroblasts discovered by Kazutoshi Takahashi at Kyoto University, Japan, in 2006. These iPS cells were already discussed in Part II. However this technology is still not clinically relevant yet, has many side effects and is not the focus of this book. [PMID37678976, PMID38069252, PMID34668236]

Nevertheless a chimeric approach of adult MSCs and iPSCs may be of clinical focus in serious diseases such as diabetes type 1 or kidney failure. [PMID35386912, PMID24515922]

In addition as discussed below, a major focus of Regenerative Medicine will be "cell-free" stem cell preparations including ECM and exosomes as discussed below. In addition, there are regenerative effects in many other synthetic compounds such as peptides and hyaluronic acid.

This book concentrates on the realistic and ethically viable options in regenerative medicine, highlighting the significant advancements made with adult stem cells. While acknowledging the historical context and scientific value of embryonic and fetal stem cell research, our focus remains firmly on the practical and rapidly advancing field of 'adult stem cell' therapy. This approach aligns with the current trends in medical research and public ethical standards, ensuring that the information provided is both relevant and responsible.

MSCs - what can they do?

Multipotent mesenchymal stromal cells (MSCs), often referred to as mesenchymal stem cells, are a type of adult stem cell with significant potential in regenerative medicine due to their ability to differentiate into a variety of cell types and their powerful immunomodulatory effects. Here's a comprehensive overview of MSCs, their sources, capabilities, and limitations:

Sources of MSCs

Bone Marrow: Bone marrow is one of the most traditional sources of MSCs. These cells play a key role in the marrow microenvironment, supporting hematopoiesis and maintaining bone homeostasis.

Umbilical Cord: The Wharton's jelly of the umbilical cord is rich in MSCs. These cells are particularly valued for their higher proliferation rates and lower immunogenicity compared to bone marrow-derived MSCs.

Adipose Tissue: Adipose-derived stem cells (ASCs) are another abundant source of MSCs. They are easier to harvest in large quantities and with minimal discomfort compared to bone marrow aspiration.

Other Tissues: MSCs can also be isolated from other tissues including dental pulp, peripheral blood, fallopian tube, and placenta, each source potentially influencing the cell's properties and therapeutic potential.

Capabilities of MSCs

Differentiation: MSCs are multipotent, meaning they can differentiate into osteoblasts (bone cells), chondrocytes (cartilage cells), myocytes (muscle cells), and adipocytes (fat cells), among others. This differentiation capacity is crucial for applications in tissue repair and regeneration.

Immunomodulation: MSCs can modulate immune responses by interacting with various immune cells. They can inhibit T cell proliferation, modulate B cells, and affect the function of natural killer cells and dendritic cells. This makes them promising for treating autoimmune diseases and for use in organ transplantation.

Secretion of Paracrine Factors: MSCs release cytokines and growth factors that help modulate the local tissue environment, promoting healing and suppressing inflammatory responses. This paracrine activity is often considered more significant than their differentiation capability in mediating therapeutic effects.

Limitations of MSCs

Finite Life Cycle: MSCs can only undergo a limited number of cell divisions before they enter a state known as senescence. This limits their long-term expansion and utility in clinical applications.

Restricted Differentiation: While MSCs are multipotent, they are not pluripotent like embryonic stem cells and thus have a more limited range of differentiation.

Variability: MSCs from different sources may exhibit significant variability in their efficacy, phenotype, and differentiation potential. Even MSCs from the same source but different donors can show considerable variability in their biological properties.

In conclusion, multipotent mesenchymal stromal cells (MSCs) are a cornerstone of current clinical regenerative medicine, offering diverse therapeutic potentials due to their ability to differentiate into several cell types, modulate immune responses, and secrete beneficial paracrine factors. In fact, their clinical application is nuanced due to their finite life cycle, restricted differentiation capacity, and variability depending on the source and extraction method. Ongoing research aims to optimize their use, enhance their therapeutic potential, and overcome the limitations associated with their senescence and source-dependent variability.

To summarize, multipotent mesenchymal stromal cells (MSCs) are 'adult stem cells' and further progressed. They can be isolated from various tissues such as bone marrow and umbilical cord. They have a finite life cycle and restricted ability to differentiate further.

The Functional Dynamics of Mesenchymal Stem Cells (MSCs)

Lets go deeper into the question of what are MSCs and what do MSCs actually do in the body? In this section, we delve into the scientific underpinnings of mesenchymal stem cells (MSCs) and their therapeutic actions. Before exploring the intricate details, here's a brief overview of the key functions and mechanisms through which MSCs contribute to regenerative medicine and healing:

Reduction of general Inflammation:

Interleukins: MSCs play a crucial role in modulating the immune system. MSCs release anti-inflammatory molecules, including various interleukins, which help in reducing inflammation. This property is particularly beneficial in treating conditions where inflammation is a primary concern, such as autoimmune diseases and inflammatory arthritis. Interleukins are a major player in controlling inflammation, however there are many more discussed below. [PMID38886861]

Reduction of Scar Tissue:

MicroRNA and Healing: MSCs are involved in tissue repair and reducing scar formation, partly due to their secretion of specific microRNAs. These microRNAs can regulate gene expression in the damaged tissues, promoting healing and reducing fibrosis, which is the formation of scar tissue.

Homing and Differentiation:

Chemokines and Growth Factors: MSCs have the ability to 'home' to sites of injury or damage, a process guided by chemokines – signaling proteins released by damaged tissues. Once at the injury site, MSCs can differentiate into various cell types under the influence of local growth factors. This differentiation is crucial in repairing and regenerating damaged tissues.

Direction of New Tissue Formation:

Cartilage and Other Tissues: MSCs can direct the formation of new tissues, including cartilage, which is particularly relevant in conditions like osteoarthritis. They can also recruit the body's own stem cells, such as pericytes (cells found in small blood vessels), to participate in the repair and regeneration process.

Recruiting the Body's own Stem Cells:

Pericytes and Regeneration: By recruiting pericytes and other resident stem cells, MSCs can amplify the regenerative process, facilitating the repair of damaged tissues and the formation of new, healthy tissue.

These are the most important steps in the possible functionality of MSCs, however not necessarily in this order! Keep in mind that research science on the topic of MSCs and their function is very active and some major discoveries may still lie ahead of us.

Now we will provide a more detailed examination of these aspects of MSCs. As we proceed to a more In-Depth Exploration, we will focus on these mechanisms of action:

1. Understanding the complex interactions and signaling pathways involved in MSC function.

2. Clinical Implications: How these mechanisms translate into therapeutic potential for various diseases.

3. Research and Developments: Current research findings that elucidate the role of MSCs in regenerative medicine.

4. Therapeutic Challenges and Future Directions: Addressing the challenges in harnessing MSCs for therapy and the future directions in MSC research.

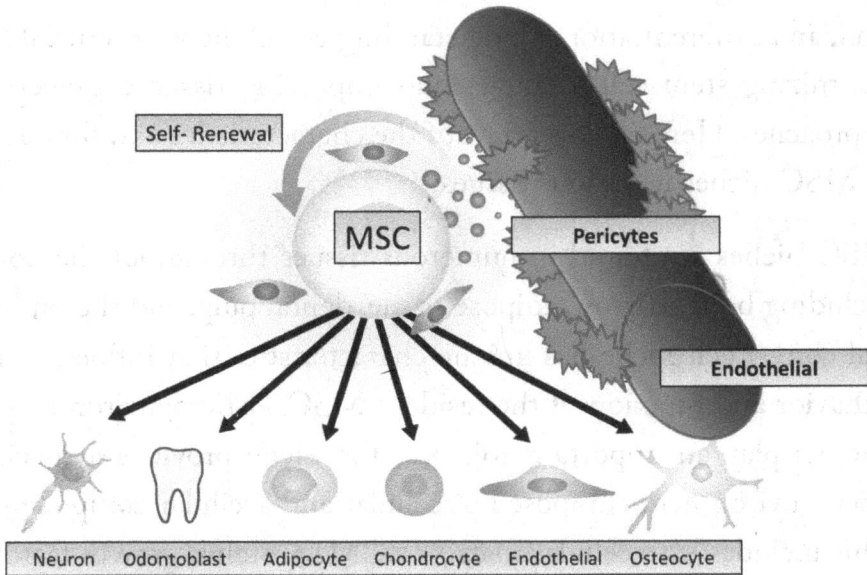

Fig. 8: MSCs have a limited ability to reproduce and differentiate into various tissues. They reside in niches, such as those provided by pericytes on arterial walls.

"The Stem Cell Extracellular Matrix"

The MSCs 'Niche' and What Maintains Its Balance

Mesenchymal stem cells (MSCs) reside in specialized microenvironments within various tissues, known as stem cell niches. These niches provide a critical support system that maintains MSCs in an undifferentiated and self-renewable state, and they play a key role in regulating the balance between stem cell quiescence, proliferation, and differentiation. Understanding MSC niches is crucial for optimizing stem cell therapies and improving tissue engineering approaches. Here's an overview of the characteristics and functions of MSC niches in various tissues:

MSC niches are found in numerous tissues throughout the body, including bone marrow, adipose tissue, dental pulp, and the umbilical cord. Each niche has unique characteristics that influence the behavior and function of the resident MSCs. Microenvironmental Factors play an important role and the niche provides a specific microenvironment composed of cellular and acellular components. This includes extracellular matrix (ECM) proteins, growth factors, and cytokines that interact with MSCs to regulate their fate. MSCs in their niches interact with various cell types, including immune cells, endothelial cells, and other stem cells. These interactions are crucial for maintaining MSC properties and responding to physiological demands.

Specific Niches and Their Functions

MSC fibroblast pluripotent stem cells live in 'stem cell niches'.

1. Bone Marrow Niche: The bone marrow is the most well-studied source of MSCs. In this niche, MSCs are primarily involved in supporting hematopoiesis (blood cell formation) and bone homeostasis. They interact closely with hematopoietic stem cells (HSCs) and are influenced by signals from endothelial cells and adipocytes within the marrow.

2. Adipose Tissue Niche: MSCs in adipose tissue, often referred to as adipose-derived stem cells (ASCs), play roles in adipogenesis and the secretion of various paracrine factors that influence immune modulation and tissue repair.

3. Dental Pulp Niche: MSCs in dental pulp (dental pulp stem cells, DPSCs) are involved in the regeneration of dentin and other dental structures. They respond to injury by differentiating into odontoblasts, which are responsible for new dentin formation.

4. Umbilical Cord Niche: MSCs derived from Wharton's jelly of the umbilical cord have potent immunomodulatory functions and are used in various therapeutic applications. The umbilical cord niche is particularly rich in hyaluronic acid, which supports the expansion and function of MSCs.

Therapeutic Implications and Challenges

- Therapeutic Use: Leveraging the regenerative and immuno-modulatory capabilities of MSCs from these niches has led to treatments for a range of disorders, including autoimmune diseases, degenerative diseases, and injuries.

- Challenges in Clinical Use: A major challenge is maintaining the 'stemness' and functional properties of MSCs once they are removed from their niche for clinical use. The niche-specific signals are often lost in culture, which can affect the efficacy of MSC-based therapies.

- Niche Mimicking in Tissue Engineering: Advances in tissue engineering aim to recreate aspects of the MSC niche in vitro to maintain and enhance the therapeutic properties of MSCs. This includes the development of biomaterials that mimic the natural ECM and the incorporation of growth factors and cytokines that are present in the niche.

MSC niches are vital for maintaining the properties of stem cells and understanding these niches is crucial for harnessing the potential of MSCs in regenerative medicine. Ongoing research focuses on better understanding these environments and how they can be mimicked or preserved during MSC expansion and application in therapies.

MSCs can self-renew for a limited number of times and differentiate into multiple tissues. From tissue cultures we know that within 43 to 77 days (7 to 12 passages) they undergo senescence. [PMID18493317]

As the body ages, changes in the stem cell niches, including those that house mesenchymal stem cells (MSCs), are a significant factor contributing to the decline in regenerative capacity observed in elderly individuals. These changes impact the functionality, availability, and behavior of MSCs. Here's an overview of how aging affects MSC niches and the implications of these changes:

Age-Related Changes in MSC Niches

Decreased MSC Numbers: Studies have shown that the number of functional MSCs in various tissues declines with age. This reduction in stem cell numbers can be attributed to several factors, including a decrease in the regenerative potential of the niche environments. Estimates are that from age 10 to 60 we have 1000 time less msc

Altered Niche Functionality: Aging can alter the cellular composition and the extracellular matrix (ECM) within the niches. Changes in the ECM components, such as increased fibrosis or altered integrin signaling, can disrupt the interactions between MSCs and their niche, affecting MSC maintenance and function.

Reduced Responsiveness to Signals: Aged MSCs often exhibit reduced responsiveness to growth factors and cytokines that are crucial for their activation and differentiation. This can lead to impaired regenerative responses and slower healing processes.

Senescence of MSCs: MSCs in older individuals are more likely to enter a state of senescence, characterized by a cessation of cell division and alterations in secreted factors. Senescent MSCs can secrete pro-inflammatory cytokines, contributing to the age-related increase in systemic inflammation, known as "inflammaging."

Implications for Regenerative Medicine

We have already shown you in Fig. 3 how drastically MSC function reduces with age. Unfortunately this presents an argument against using autologous MSCs at least for now. A better understanding of the regenerative stem cell niches may change this in the future.

Therapeutic Efficacy: The age-related decline in MSC functionality can affect the efficacy of autologous MSC therapies, where patients' own cells are used for treatment. Older patients' MSCs may not be as effective in regenerative therapies due to these changes.

Donor Age Considerations: In treatments involving allogeneic MSCs, where cells are sourced from donors, the age of the donor can be an important factor in determining the therapeutic potential of the harvested cells.

Strategies to Counteract Aging Effects- Enhancing Niche Environment:

Strategies to rejuvenate the stem cell niche or to mimic the young niche environment in vitro can help maintain or restore the functionality of aged MSCs. This includes using scaffolds and hydrogels that replicate the young ECM or administering compounds that reverse senescent states.

Preconditioning MSCs: Preconditioning or priming MSCs through exposure to certain growth factors, hypoxic conditions, or pharmacological agents before application may enhance their regenerative capabilities and resilience.

Selective Cell Expansion: Techniques to selectively expand more potent subpopulations of MSCs that retain their functionality despite the aging process could improve outcomes in regenerative medicine applications.

Tissue	Number of Stem Cells (Young Age)	Age-Related Loss	Number of Stem Cells (Old Age)
Hair Follicles	High	Significant decline	Low
Gut Epithelium	Very High	Moderate decline	Moderate to Low
Heart	Low	Minimal decline	Very Low
Lung	Moderate	Moderate decline	Low
Bone Marrow	High	Significant decline	Low
Liver	Moderate	Moderate decline	Low to Moderate
Kidney	Low	Moderate decline	Very Low
Brain	Low	Moderate decline	Very Low

Table 2: Comparison of relative decline of stem cell numbers at younger vs. older age (varies by individual)

Age-Related Stem cell loss:

Hair Follicles: Stem cells in hair follicles decline significantly with age, leading to thinning hair and baldness.

Gut Epithelium: The gut epithelium has a high turnover rate with moderate stem cell loss over time, impacting gut health.

Heart: Cardiac stem cells are limited and show minimal regenerative capacity, which declines further with age. Lung: Lung stem cells decrease moderately, affecting the lung's ability to repair and regenerate.

Bone Marrow: Hematopoietic stem cells in the bone marrow decline significantly, reducing the body's ability to produce new blood cells.

Liver: Hepatic stem cells have a moderate decline, which can impair the liver's regenerative capacity.

Kidney: Renal stem cells are few and their numbers decline moderately, leading to decreased kidney repair capability.

Brain: Neural stem cells are limited and decline with age, contributing to cognitive decline and neurodegenerative diseases.

In conclusion, the number of stem cells in various tissues declines with age, affecting the body's ability to regenerate and repair tissues. Understanding these changes is crucial for developing age-related therapeutic strategies. Aging has a profound impact on MSC niches, reducing the number and functional capacity of MSCs and affecting their ability to contribute to tissue repair. Understanding and mitigating the effects of aging on MSCs and their niches is critical for advancing regenerative therapies, particularly for older patients. This involves both improving our understanding of niche biology and developing advanced biotechnological interventions to enhance stem cell functionality. For this reason umbilical cord sources are considered richest in numbers for both clinical and research purposes.

The Role of the Extracellular Matrix (ECM)

In order to understand the topic of 'cellular matrix', let us dive a little deeper into the science of cell-cell interactions. The statement

"No eukaryotic cell is happy on its own" highlights the fundamental differences between eukaryotic and prokaryotic cells in terms of their requirements for growth and survival. Here's a closer look at these differences:

Eukaryotic Cells in Tissue Culture: The general consensus is that human eukaryotic cells (cells with a distinct nucleus) have a need to either be attached to a matrix or to another cell that is neighboring them. In tissue culture single cells have low survival rate and cannot typically be suspended in solution for very long times.

Surface Attachment:

Eukaryotic cells, such as human cells, typically require attachment to a specific surface to grow and survive in vitro. This surface can be the bottom of a tissue culture dish coated with proteins like collagen, fibronectin, or laminin, which facilitate cell adhesion.

Cell-Cell Interactions:

In addition to surface attachment, eukaryotic cells often need to interact with each other to maintain their health and function. These interactions can be mediated through cell junctions, extracellular matrix components, and paracrine signaling.

Extracellular Matrix (ECM):

The ECM plays a crucial role in providing structural support and biochemical cues to eukaryotic cells. It influences cell behavior, including proliferation, differentiation, and migration.

Growth Factors and Nutrients: Eukaryotic cells in tissue culture require a nutrient-rich medium supplemented with growth factors and other essential molecules to support their metabolic needs and growth.

In contrast, Prokaryotic Cells can be alive for long periods separated in Liquid Suspension due to their rigid cell wall:

Prokaryotic cells (cells without a nucleus), such as E. coli, have a strong cell wall that provides structural integrity and protection. This allows them to thrive in a variety of environments, including liquid suspensions, without the need for surface attachment.

Growth in Suspension: Prokaryotic cells can grow and divide rapidly in liquid culture media, as they can absorb nutrients directly from their surroundings and do not rely on surface attachment or complex cell-cell interactions.

Simpler Requirements: Compared to eukaryotic cells, prokaryotic cells have simpler growth requirements and can often be cultured in relatively simple media, making them easier to grow in the laboratory.

Why is this important?

The need for cell stability means that the extracellular matrix (ECM) in birth tissue-derived mesenchymal stem cells (MSCs) plays a crucial role in maintaining the structural and functional integrity of tissues. Birth tissues, such as the placenta, umbilical cord, and amniotic membrane, are rich sources of MSCs, and their ECM components contribute significantly to the regenerative properties of these cells. Here's an overview of the ECM in birth tissue MSCs:

Subtitle: Extracellular Matrix from Birth Tissue

Birth tissues comprising umbilical cord, placenta and amniotic fluid are rich in Extracellular Matrix molecules. Naturally MSC preparations from these tissues bring with them this important structural component. These ECMs allow for the following functions:

Supporting Cell Structure: The ECM provides a scaffold that supports the physical structure of the tissue and maintains the proper organization of cells.

Regulating Cell Behavior: Components of the ECM interact with cell surface receptors to influence cell behavior, including adhesion, migration, proliferation, and differentiation.

Facilitating Cell Communication:

The ECM acts as a reservoir for signaling molecules, facilitating communication between cells and their microenvironment.

Modulating Immune Responses: The ECM in birth tissue MSCs can modulate immune responses, contributing to the immunomodulatory properties of these cells.

Promoting Tissue Regeneration: The unique composition of the ECM in birth tissue MSCs supports tissue regeneration and repair, making these cells promising candidates for regenerative medicine applications.

Some regenerative products are simply providing just ECM without live MSCs in assisting a healing process. Hyaluronic acid and glycosaminoglycans are well known simple key ingredients that are effective especially in cosmetic applications.

ECM constituents:

In more detail, the ECM of birth tissue contains many constituents. Here are a few players that concern us:

Collagen: Collagen is a major component of the ECM in birth tissue MSCs, providing structural support and strength to the tissue. It plays a vital role in cell adhesion, migration, and differentiation.

Fibronectin: Fibronectin is a glycoprotein involved in cell adhesion and migration. It also plays a role in wound healing and tissue repair processes.

Hyaluronic Acid: Hyaluronic acid is a glycosaminoglycan that provides hydration and lubrication to the ECM. It is particularly abundant in the Wharton's jelly of the umbilical cord, contributing to its viscoelastic properties.

Proteoglycans: Proteoglycans are important for maintaining the hydration and resilience of the ECM. They also play a role in modulating cell signaling pathways.

Growth Factors and Cytokines

The extracellular matrix (ECM) of birth tissue MSCs is rich in various growth factors and cytokines that are crucial for cell proliferation, differentiation, and tissue regeneration. These components create a supportive environment for MSCs and enhance their regenerative capabilities. Key growth factors and cytokines present in the ECM of birth tissue MSCs include:

- Vascular Endothelial Growth Factor (VEGF): Promotes angiogenesis and blood vessel formation.

- Transforming Growth Factor-Beta (TGF-β): Regulates cell growth, differentiation, and immune response.

- Fibroblast Growth Factor (FGF): Stimulates cell proliferation and differentiation.

- Epidermal Growth Factor (EGF): Promotes cell growth and differentiation.

- Platelet-Derived Growth Factor (PDGF): Regulates cell growth and division.

- Insulin-Like Growth Factor (IGF): Stimulates growth and development.

- Interleukin-10 (IL-10): Anti-inflammatory cytokine that reduces inflammation and promotes healing.

- Interleukin-4 (IL-4): Anti-inflammatory cytokine that supports immune modulation and tissue repair.

These bioactive molecules play significant roles in mediating the beneficial effects of MSCs in tissue repair and regeneration, making the ECM of birth tissue MSCs a powerful tool in regenerative medicine.

In summary, the extracellular matrix of birth tissue-derived MSCs is a complex and dynamic component that plays a critical role [PMID22267536] in the regenerative and therapeutic potential of these cells. Understanding the composition and functions of the ECM in these tissues is essential for harnessing their full potential in regenerative medicine and tissue engineering. This may be an important factor in wound healing as well. [PMID37867186]

In addition, the extracellular matrix (ECM) plays a pivotal role in maintaining the stability and viability of eukaryotic cells in tissue culture and during cryopreservation. Here's how ECM contributes to cell stability in these conditions:

ECM - Importance in Tissue Culture

Many autologously harvested stem cell fractions can be grown in tissue culture for the purpose of multiplication or research. It is crucial that ECM as well as proper medium is provided for this process. The ECM delivers a variety of very important longevity factors.

Structural Support: The ECM provides a scaffold that supports cell adhesion, spreading, and organization. This structural support is crucial for maintaining the integrity and morphology of cells in culture.

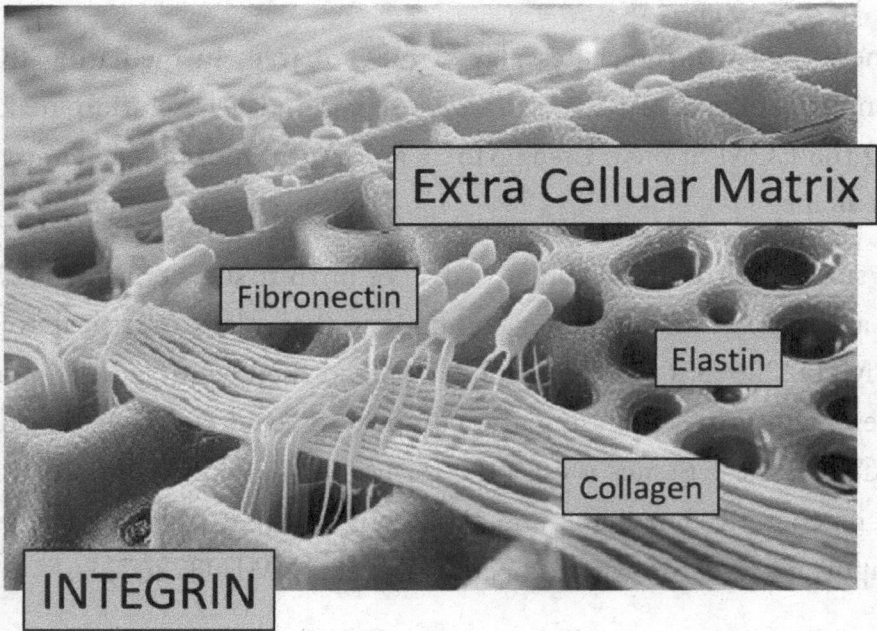

Fig.9: Extracellular matrix (ECM) is a mesh of extracellular macro-molecules and minerals, such as collagen, enzymes and glycoproteins; this structure is crucial for the stability of cells. Integrins are important receptors in the cell membrane required to bind protein filaments in the cytoplasm and the ECM

Cell-ECM Interactions: Cell surface receptors, such as integrins, interact with ECM components like collagen, fibronectin, and

128

laminin. These interactions are essential for cell survival, proliferation, and differentiation.

Mimicking the Natural Environment: In vitro, the ECM can be used to recreate aspects of the cells' natural environment, promoting more physiologically relevant behavior and responses.

Regulation of Signaling Pathways: The ECM modulates various signaling pathways that are critical for cell growth, metabolism, and gene expression.

The extracellular matrix (ECM) is a crucial component of the cellular microenvironment, providing structural support and biochemical cues that influence cell behavior. In tissue culture, mimicking the ECM is essential for maintaining cell function and promoting specific cellular responses. Here's how the ECM is mimicked in tissue culture dishes:

Coating dish surfaces with ECM Proteins

Collagen: Collagen is a major component of the ECM and is commonly used to coat tissue culture dishes. It provides a natural substrate for cell adhesion and supports cell proliferation and differentiation.

Fibronectin: Fibronectin is another ECM protein that promotes cell adhesion, spreading, and migration. Coating dishes with fibronectin can enhance the attachment of cells that express fibronectin receptors.

Laminin: Laminin is important for basement membrane formation and is used to coat culture dishes for cells that require this specific ECM component, such as epithelial and neuronal cells.

Gelatin: Gelatin, derived from collagen, is a less expensive alternative used for coating dishes. It provides a simple adhesive surface for a variety of cell types.

Synthetic and Natural Hydrogels

Matrigel: Matrigel is a commercially available gelatinous protein mixture derived from the ECM of mouse tumor cells. It contains laminin, collagen, and growth factors, providing a complex ECM environment for cell culture.

Agarose and Alginate: Agarose and alginate are natural polysaccharides used to create hydrogels that mimic the ECM's physical properties. They provide a three-dimensional scaffold for cell culture, particularly for tissue engineering applications.

Synthetic Hydrogels: Synthetic hydrogels, such as polyethylene glycol (PEG)-based hydrogels, can be chemically modified to incorporate cell-adhesive peptides and growth factors, offering customizable ECM-like environments. [PMID38334602]

Micro- and Nanofabrication Techniques

Micropatterning: Micropatterning techniques, such as photolithography, can create defined patterns of ECM proteins on culture dishes, allowing for the control of cell shape, orientation, and organization.

Nanofibers: Electrospun nanofibers made from biodegradable polymers can mimic the fibrous structure of the ECM, providing a scaffold for cell attachment and growth.

Mimicking the ECM in tissue culture dishes involves the use of ECM proteins, hydrogels, and micro- and nanofabrication techniques to create a supportive and instructive environment for cells.

These approaches enable researchers to study cell behavior in a more physiologically relevant context and are essential for the development of tissue-engineered constructs and regenerative medicine applications.

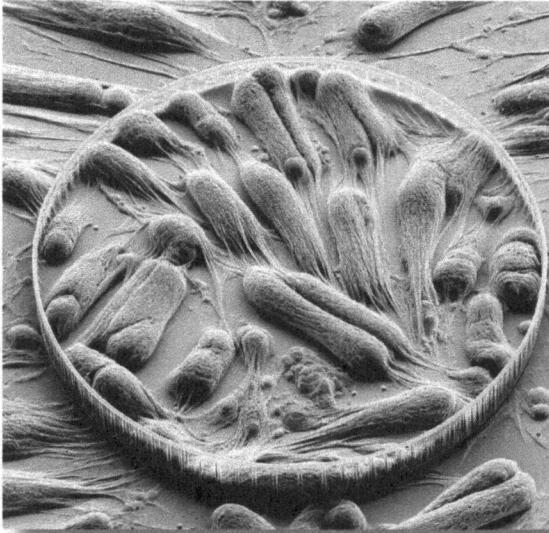

Fig.10: Cell culture of fibroblast show how individual cells are attached to the prepared surface of the dish and also to themselves

ECM and Cryopreservation

Freezing 'live cells' is actually not a trivial problem since the eukaryotic cell membrane is fragile and can easily rupture. Even the shrinkage of the cell can result in apoptotic signals. For this reason both glycerol and DMSO (Dimethyl sulfoxide) are added to the cell culture before freezing. This is called cryo-protection.

The viability of cryopreserved fibroblasts after thawing can vary depending on several factors, including the cryopreservation protocol, the concentration of dimethyl sulfoxide (DMSO) used, the freezing and thawing rates, and the handling techniques. However, under optimal conditions, the average viability of fibroblasts after thawing is typically reported to be around 70% to 90%.

Factors Affecting Viability

DMSO Concentration: DMSO is a commonly used cryoprotectant that helps protect cells from damage during the freezing and thawing process. The concentration of DMSO is critical; it is usually used at a final concentration of 5-10% for fibroblast cryopreservation.

Freezing Rate: The rate at which cells are frozen is important for maintaining viability. A controlled rate of cooling, typically around -1°C per minute, is often used to ensure optimal cell survival.

Thawing Rate: Rapid thawing is generally recommended to minimize the formation of ice crystals, which can damage cells. Thawing at 37°C in a water bath is a common practice.

Post-Thaw Handling: Careful handling of thawed cells, including the timely removal of DMSO and gentle washing, is essential to maintain viability and promote recovery.

The average viability of cryopreserved fibroblasts after thawing in the presence of DMSO is generally high, but it can be influenced by various factors related to the cryopreservation and thawing protocols. Optimizing these conditions is crucial for ensuring the maximum viability and functionality of fibroblasts for research and clinical applications.

Cryopreservation techniques for biological samples, including cells and tissues, have evolved significantly over time. The introduction of new slow liquid nitrogen (LN2) freezing machines represents an advancement in this field, offering several benefits compared to traditional flash freezing methods:

Slow-time LN2 Freezing Machines

A novel approach to keeping 'live cells' alive is the slowed down process to get down to -196 celsius (the temperature of frozen liquid nitrogen). Traditionally, flash freezing was used however this process can cause ice crystals which can destroy the structure of the cellular membrane.

Controlled Rate Freezing: Slow LN2 machines allow for precise control over the freezing rate, which is crucial for minimizing the formation of ice crystals that can damage cellular structures. A controlled rate of cooling (typically -1°C to -3°C per minute) is often optimal for preserving cell viability.

Uniform Cooling: These machines provide uniform cooling, ensuring that all parts of the sample are frozen at the same rate. This consistency reduces the risk of thermal gradients that can lead to uneven freezing and potential cell damage.

Programmable Freezing Profiles: Slow LN2 machines often come with programmable features that allow users to set specific freezing profiles tailored to the requirements of different cell types or tissues. This flexibility enhances the versatility of the machine for various applications.

Reduced Risk of Contamination: The closed system of slow LN2 machines reduces the risk of contamination compared to open-system flash freezing methods. This is particularly important for samples intended for clinical or therapeutic use.

Flash Freezing Flash freezing, such as plunge freezing in liquid nitrogen, results in rapid cooling of the sample. While this can be beneficial for certain applications, such as preserving the ultrastructure of tissues for electron microscopy, it may not be ideal for preserving cell viability.

Ice Crystal Formation: The rapid cooling rate in flash freezing can lead to the formation of large ice crystals, which can disrupt cellular membranes and organelles, leading to reduced cell viability.

Limited Control: Flash freezing offers limited control over the cooling rate and temperature, making it less suitable for samples that require precise freezing conditions.

In summary, the relatively new 'slow LN2 machines' offer several advantages over traditional flash freezing methods, particularly for the cryopreservation of cells and tissues where maintaining viability is crucial. The controlled rate freezing, uniform cooling, and programmable profiles provided by these machines enhance the preservation of biological samples, making them valuable tools in research, biobanking, and clinical applications.

Glycerol vs. DMSO as cryo-preservative

While glycerol is an effective cryoprotectant that can maintain the viability of cryopreserved fibroblasts, its effectiveness can vary based on the cryopreservation conditions, including glycerol concentration, cooling and thawing rates, and post-thaw handling. The choice between glycerol and DMSO or the decision to use them in combination depends on the specific requirements of the cell type being preserved and the goals of the cryopreservation process.

Toxicity: Glycerol is generally less toxic than DMSO, making it a preferred choice for certain applications where DMSO's cytotoxic effects are a concern.

Penetration: Glycerol penetrates cell membranes more slowly than DMSO. This slower penetration rate can be advantageous or disadvantageous, depending on the specific requirements of the cryopreservation process.

Use in Combination: In some protocols, glycerol and DMSO are used in combination to take advantage of the protective effects of both cryoprotectants.

When choosing a frozen stem cell preparation as treatment option, the choice of glycerol vs DMSO may come down to an allergy named sulfa-allergy.

Glycerol: Glycerol is an alternative cryoprotectant that does not contain sulfur and is generally well-tolerated. It is often used at concentrations of 10-15% for cryopreservation.

DMSO: excellent cell penetration and cryoprotective properties. However, it can cause allergic reactions or sensitivities in some individuals.

Side Effects: While DMSO can be beneficial, it can also cause side effects such as skin irritation, garlic-like taste and odor, and in rare cases, allergic reactions. While a sulfa allergy does not directly imply an allergy to DMSO, patients with multiple drug allergies or sensitivities may be more cautious about using DMSO-containing preparations.

Regulatory Approval: It's important to note that the use of DMSO for joint injections is not universally approved by regulatory agencies like the FDA. Its use in this context may be considered off-label or experimental, depending on the jurisdiction.

Clinical Evidence: The clinical evidence supporting the use of DMSO for joint injections is currently limited, and more research is needed to fully understand its efficacy and safety for this application. In summary, for patients with a known sulfa allergy or sensitivity to DMSO, glycerol can be a suitable alternative for stem cell cryopreservation

Clinical Considerations

Allergy Testing: If there is concern about a potential allergic reaction to DMSO, allergy testing or consultation with an allergist may be recommended before proceeding with stem cell therapy.

Informed Consent: Patients should be informed about the cryoprotectants used in their stem cell preparation and any potential risks associated with them, including allergic reactions.

Alternative Cryoprotectants: In addition to glycerol, other cryoprotectants, such as trehalose or ethylene glycol, may be considered based on the specific requirements of the stem cell type and the patient's medical history in the future.

Dimethyl sulfoxide (DMSO) is a chemical compound that has been used for various medical applications, including as a solvent for pharmaceuticals and as a topical analgesic and anti-inflammatory agent. In the context of joint injections, DMSO has been explored for its potential medicinal properties:

Anti-inflammatory Properties

Inflammation Reduction: DMSO has been shown to possess anti-inflammatory properties, which can be beneficial in reducing joint inflammation and swelling associated with conditions like osteoarthritis or rheumatoid arthritis.

Analgesic Properties

Pain Relief: DMSO has analgesic properties that can help alleviate joint pain. It is thought to work by blocking pain signals in peripheral nerves.

Enhanced Drug Delivery: DMSO can act as a solvent and carrier for other therapeutic agents, potentially enhancing their delivery and effectiveness when injected into the joint.

Antioxidant Effects: Free Radical Scavenging: DMSO has antioxidant properties, which can help reduce oxidative stress in the joint and protect against tissue damage.

In summary, Glycerol may be the safer option for some patients but DMSO has potential medicinal properties that could be beneficial for joint injections, including anti-inflammatory and analgesic effects. However, further research is necessary to establish its safety and effectiveness for treating joint conditions. As with any medical treatment, the use of DMSO for joint injections should be discussed with a healthcare professional to weigh the potential benefits and risks. Elliott 2024 recently concluded: "Due to the inherent heterogeneity in MSC populations from different sources there is still no standardized procedure for their isolation, identification, functional characterization, cryopreservation, and route of administration, and not likely to be a "one-size-fits-all" approach in their applications in cell-based therapy and regenerative medicine." [PMID38340887]

The ECM plays an important role in the cryo-protection of live cells

Most 'minimally manipulated' birth tissue MSC preparations need to be cryo-preserved (properly frozen) immediately. Once again the ECM is an important ingredient in this process.

- Protection During Freezing: The ECM can provide a protective barrier around cells during the freezing process, reducing the risk of ice crystal formation and mechanical damage to the cell membrane.

- Maintenance of Cell Structure: By preserving the structural integrity of cells, the ECM helps maintain cell viability and function upon thawing.

- Cryoprotectant Carrier: The ECM can act as a carrier for cryoprotectants, which are substances that protect cells from freezing-induced damage. The ECM can help distribute cryoprotectants evenly around the cells, enhancing their protective effects.

- Reducing Oxidative Stress: The ECM can also play a role in reducing oxidative stress during the freezing and thawing process, which is important for preserving cell viability.

The extracellular matrix is a critical component in tissue culture and cryopreservation, providing structural support, facilitating cell-ECM interactions, and modulating signaling pathways. In cryopreservation, the ECM contributes to the protection of cells during freezing, maintenance of cell structure, and reduction of oxidative stress, all of which are essential for preserving cell viability and function.

Exosomes and Secretomes

The future of stem cells: as an emerging alternative, "cell-free" stem cell products have become an option. They are easier to handle for clinical applications and more stable. These so-called 'secretome' preparations of MSC tissue cultures and birth tissues contain mostly exosomes and proteins, which are small extracellular vesicles secreted by MSC cells. Exosomes are generally more stable during cryopreservation compared to whole cells or may not need to be frozen at all. This increased stability is due to their small size, lipid bilayer structure, and lack of cellular organelles, which make them less susceptible to damage from ice crystal formation and osmotic stress during freezing and thawing.

Lipid Bilayer: The lipid bilayer of exosomes provides a protective barrier that helps maintain their integrity during the freezing and thawing process.

Small Size: The small size of exosomes (typically 30-150 nm in diameter) reduces the likelihood of mechanical damage during cryopreservation.

Cryoprotectants: Nevertheless the use of cryoprotectants such as DMSO or glycerol can further enhance the stability of exosomes during cryopreservation by preventing ice crystal formation and reducing osmotic stress.

Optimized Protocols: Developing optimized protocols for the concentration, freezing, and storage of exosomal preparations can further improve their stability during cryopreservation.

Applications for Cryopreserved Exosomes

The ability to easily cryopreserve exosomes with high stability is valuable for various applications, including:

Biomedical Research: Cryopreserved exosomes can be used as a source of biomarkers for disease diagnosis and monitoring, as well as for studying intercellular communication.

Therapeutic Use: Exosomes have potential as therapeutic agents for regenerative medicine, drug delivery, and immunomodulation. Stable cryopreservation allows for the long-term storage and transport of exosome-based therapeutics.

Clinical Trials: The stability of exosomes in cryopreservation facilitates their use in clinical trials, where consistent and reproducible exosome preparations are required.

In contrast to 'live cells', Exosomes exhibit good stability during cryopreservation, making them suitable for long-term storage and use in various biomedical applications. Optimizing cryopreservation protocols and the use of appropriate cryoprotectants can further enhance the stability and integrity of exosomal preparations.

Integrins: Key Receptors in ECM-Stem Cell Interactions

The ECM has many components as mentioned above, however 'Integrins' are worth giving a special introduction here. They play a crucial role in the interactions between stem cells and the extracellular matrix (ECM), influencing various cellular processes essential for tissue homeostasis and repair. Here's an overview of how integrins mediate ECM-stem cell interactions:

Structure and Function: Integrins are transmembrane receptors (see Fig. 9 above) composed of alpha and beta subunits. They facilitate cell-ECM adhesion by binding to specific ECM components such as fibronectin, collagen, and laminin.

Adhesion and Anchorage: Integrins are critical for the adhesion of stem cells to the ECM. This adhesion is essential for maintaining stem cell niches, where stem cells reside in a specific anatomic location within the tissue. The anchorage provided by integrins is crucial for stem cell survival, as it prevents 'anoikis' (a form of programmed cell death induced by detachment from the ECM).

Homing and Migration: Integrins play a vital role in the homing of stem cells to sites of injury or inflammation. They mediate the migration of stem cells by interacting with the ECM, guiding the cells to their target locations for tissue repair.

Signal Transduction: Upon binding to ECM components, integrins activate various intracellular signaling pathways that regulate stem cell proliferation, differentiation, and self-renewal.

These signals are essential for the proper functioning of stem cells and their ability to respond to environmental cues.

The Role of Omega-3 in ECM Stiffness and Stem Cell Differentiation

Regulation of Stem Cell Fate:

The interaction between integrins and the ECM can influence stem cell fate decisions. For example, the stiffness of the ECM, which is sensed by integrins, can dictate whether stem cells differentiate into specific cell types.

Omega-3 fatty acids, particularly docosahexaenoic acid (DHA), play a significant role in modulating the stiffness of the extracellular matrix (ECM). This modulation is crucial as it impacts how integrins, which are transmembrane receptors on the cell surface, sense the mechanical properties of the ECM. The stiffness of the ECM, influenced by its lipid composition, including omega-3 fatty acids, can dictate the differentiation pathways of stem cells, steering them towards specific cell types.

ECM Stiffness and Cell Differentiation:

Soft ECM: A softer ECM environment, often associated with higher omega-3 content, tends to support the differentiation of stem cells into adipogenic (fat) cells. This is because the increased membrane fluidity provided by omega-3 fatty acids makes the ECM less rigid.

Stiff ECM: Conversely, a stiffer ECM, typically resulting from lower omega-3 content, encourages the differentiation of stem cells into osteogenic (bone) cells. The reduced flexibility and increased rigidity of the ECM provide the necessary mechanical cues for bone formation.

Integrin Signaling:

Integrins are integral in the mechanosensing of ECM properties. They detect changes in ECM stiffness and initiate intracellular signaling pathways that influence gene expression and ultimately determine cell fate. The presence of omega-3 fatty acids in the ECM affects these mechanical properties, thereby influencing integrin signaling and stem cell differentiation.

Mechanisms of Omega-3 Influence:

Incorporation into Cell Membranes: Omega-3 fatty acids, particularly DHA, are incorporated into the cell membranes, affecting their elasticity and flexibility. This incorporation is crucial for maintaining a dynamic and responsive ECM.

Adipogenesis and Osteogenesis: The presence of omega-3s in the ECM supports adipogenesis (fat cell formation) when the ECM is softer and osteogenesis (bone cell formation) when the ECM is stiffer. This differential effect underscores the importance of ECM stiffness in directing stem cell fate.

Larson 2011: "Omega-3 fatty acids modulate collagen signaling in human platelets. Collagen-mediated platelet signaling events of integrin activation, α-granule secretion, and phosphatidylserine exposure were all reduced by roughly 50% after omega-3 incorporation, and collagen-induced tyrosine phosphorylation was significantly impaired" [PMID21177087]

In conclusion, Omega-3 fatty acids significantly impact the stiffness of the ECM, which is a critical factor sensed by integrins. This mechanosensing mechanism plays a pivotal role in determining whether stem cells will differentiate into specific cell types. Understanding the influence of omega-3s on ECM properties provides valuable insights into tissue engineering and regenerative medicine, highlighting their potential in manipulating stem cell environments for desired therapeutic outcomes

Future Research and Clinical Implications on Integrins

An increasing number of studies are exploring the role of integrins in stem cell biology, with implications for tissue engineering, regenerative medicine, and cancer research.

Understanding how integrins mediate ECM-stem cell interactions can lead to the development of novel therapies that enhance tissue regeneration or target cancer stem cells. Developing Integrins for regenerative purposes without the use of live MSCs is a major focus of interest.

Here are a few noteworthy publications on this topic. Gazzato 2014 concludes "ECM represents an essential player in the stem cell niche, since it can directly or indirectly modulate the maintenance, proliferation, self-renewal and differentiation of stem cells". [PMID24418517]

Ying 2021 writes: "In this review, we summarize, for the first time, the potential mechanisms by which integrins promote MSC multilineage differentiation, including integrin downstream signaling cascades and the interactions between integrin and ion channels, the cytoskeleton, and nuclear mechanoresponses. Furthermore, we focus on the current state and future prospects of the application of integrins to promote cell differentiation." [PMID24418517]

In summary, Integrins are key receptors involved in mediating the interactions between stem cells and the extracellular matrix. They play critical roles in the adhesion, anchorage, homing, and signal transduction of stem cells, ultimately influencing stem cell fate and function. As research in this area progresses, the manipulation of integrin-ECM interactions may offer new avenues for therapeutic interventions in regenerative medicine and also cancer treatment.

Introduction to MSC Technology

Advancements and Techniques

As we already dove into some technological aspects above, it is often difficult to separate theory and practice in cellular biology. Umbilical cord is considered the richest source of MSCs [PMID26354202] and it could be argued it comes with the most regenerative message. However other sources are also viable for various reasons. This section of this book aims to provide a brief understanding of the scientific basis for the therapeutic use of different sources of MSCs and their techniques. Keep in mind this topic is usually subject to the proprietary knowledge of the manufacturers. Particularly the different effects on the immune response has to be of much future research focus. By exploring their multifaceted roles in reducing inflammation, minimizing scar tissue formation, homing to injury sites, differentiating into various cell types, and directing new tissue formation, we gain insights into the immense potential of different MSC sources in regenerative medicine.

Variability in MSC Therapies Based on Source

One of the biggest topics in Regenerative Medicine is the use of autologous vs. allogeneic stem cell sources. Here we can only briefly touch on autologous methods (harvesting one's own stem cells from bone marrow or adipose tissue).

As we delve deeper into the scientific nuances of mesenchymal stem cells (MSCs), it's crucial to bear in mind a key factor that significantly influences the outcomes and efficacy of MSC-based therapies: the source of the MSCs. The variability in the results and effectiveness of MSC therapies is often closely tied to whether the stem cells are allogeneic (donor-derived) or autologous (derived from the patient's own body).

Allogeneic vs. Autologous MSCs:

Allogeneic MSCs: These are harvested from a donor and have the advantage of being readily available for use. However, the risk of immune reaction, albeit lower than other cell types, still exists. In practice however the MSCs derived from this source are considered 'immune-privileged' if there is no contamination with other cellular tissues. Their therapeutic efficacy can vary and be influenced by the donor's characteristics, such as age and health.

Autologous MSCs: Derived from the patient's own body, these cells have a lower risk of immune rejection although some may still exist because cells are injected into different tissues elsewhere in the body. However in the clinic, after considerable manipulation this is almost never an issue. The efficacy can vary greatly depending on the patient's age, health status, and the specific tissue the MSCs are harvested from.

Influence of Source on Therapeutic Outcomes: The source of MSCs can affect their potency, differentiation capacity, and the overall therapeutic outcome. For instance, MSCs from older individuals or from certain tissues might have reduced regenerative potential.

Consistency and Standardization Challenges: Variability in the source of MSCs poses challenges in standardizing treatments and in achieving consistent results in clinical trials. This makes comparing outcomes across different studies difficult.

Ethical and Regulatory Considerations: The choice between allogeneic and autologous MSCs also brings into play different ethical and regulatory considerations, impacting the approval and application of therapies.

Personalized Approach: Understanding the variability based on MSC source is key to developing personalized treatment plans. Tailoring MSC therapies to individual patients' needs could enhance efficacy and minimize risks.

Future Research Directions: Ongoing research is focusing on understanding how the source of MSCs influences their properties and therapeutic potential. This includes exploring ways to enhance the efficacy of MSCs regardless of their origin.

Throughout the following section, we will explore these aspects in greater depth, underlining the importance of MSC source in determining the success of stem cell therapies. Recognizing this variability is essential for both researchers and clinicians in the field of regenerative medicine, as it guides the development of more effective, personalized treatments and informs the interpretation of research findings.

Autologous Bone marrow derived MSCs technique

Autologous bone marrow-derived mesenchymal stem cells (BM-MSCs) are a valuable source for regenerative medicine due to their potential to differentiate into various cell types and modulate immune responses. Here's an overview of the technique used to isolate, culture, and use autologous BM-MSCs:

Isolation of BM-MSCs

Bone Marrow Aspiration: Bone marrow is typically aspirated from the iliac crest (hip bone) under local or general anesthesia. The procedure is performed using a needle and syringe to extract a small volume of bone marrow.

Density Gradient Centrifugation: The bone marrow aspirate is then processed to isolate mononuclear cells, which include MSCs. This is often done using density gradient centrifugation, where the sample is layered over a density gradient medium and centrifuged to separate cells based on their density.

Isolation of MSCs: The mononuclear cell layer, which contains MSCs, is collected and washed to remove any remaining density gradient medium and debris.

Culture and Expansion of BM-MSCs

Seeding and Culture: The isolated mononuclear cells are seeded in culture flasks and maintained in a suitable culture medium, typically containing fetal bovine serum (FBS) and growth factors. MSCs adhere to the plastic surface of the culture flask, while non-adherent cells are removed during media changes.

Expansion: The MSCs are allowed to proliferate until they reach 70-80% confluence. At this point, they are detached using an enzymatic solution (e.g., trypsin-EDTA) and subcultured into new flasks to further expand the cell population.

Characterization: During the expansion process, the cells are monitored for their morphology, growth rate, and expression of specific surface markers (e.g., CD73, CD90, CD105) to confirm their mesenchymal stem cell identity.

Autologous Transplantation

Harvesting and Preparation: Once a sufficient number of MSCs are expanded, they are harvested and prepared for transplantation.

The cells may be concentrated and suspended in an appropriate vehicle for injection.

Transplantation: The autologous BM-MSCs are then transplanted back into the patient at the site of injury or disease. The mode of administration can vary depending on the target tissue and the clinical application (e.g., intra-articular injection for osteoarthritis, intravenous infusion for systemic conditions).

Follow-Up: Patients are monitored for any adverse reactions and followed up to assess the efficacy of the treatment in terms of symptom relief, tissue repair, and functional improvement.

The use of autologous bone marrow-derived MSCs offers a promising approach for regenerative therapies, with the advantage of being patient-specific and minimizing the risk of immune rejection. However, the technique requires careful execution at each step, from bone marrow aspiration to cell transplantation, to ensure the safety and effectiveness of the therapy and is not without side effects.

Isolation of Adipose-SVF

Stromal Vascular Fraction (SVF) derived from adipose tissue is a rich source of mesenchymal stem cells (MSCs) and other regenerative cells. The process of isolating and utilizing SVF-derived MSCs involves several steps although it can vary in different clinics and different methodologies:

Adipose Tissue Collection: Adipose tissue is typically obtained through liposuction from areas such as the abdomen, thighs, or buttocks. The procedure is usually performed under local anesthesia.

Enzymatic Digestion: The collected adipose tissue is subjected to enzymatic digestion using collagenase to break down the extracellular matrix and release the cells within the stromal vascular fraction.

Centrifugation: After digestion, the tissue suspension is centrifuged to separate the SVF, which contains MSCs, endothelial cells, pericytes, and other cell types, from the adipocytes (fat cells) and other debris.

Washing and Filtration: The SVF pellet is washed with a saline solution and filtered to remove any remaining enzymatic solution and cellular debris.

SVF Mechanical vs. Enzymatic Separation Techniques

Mechanical Separation Techniques: Centrifugation, filtration, and physical agitation depending on equipment technology

Procedure: Tissue is minced, washed, and subjected to physical forces to separate stromal vascular fraction (SVF) from adipose tissue.

- Advantages are safety: No enzymatic agents, reducing potential for contamination.

- Regulatory Approval: Easier to get regulatory approval due to the absence of enzymes.

- Cost: Lower cost due to the use of basic equipment and no need for enzymatic reagents.

- Disadvantages may be yield: Typically lower yield of SVF cells compared to enzymatic methods although this can vastly vary with the equipment used.

- Cell Viability: Mechanical forces can sometimes reduce cell viability.

Enzymatic Separation Techniques: Use of collagenase or other enzymes.

Procedure: Adipose tissue is digested with enzymes to break down the extracellular matrix, followed by centrifugation to isolate SVF cells.

- Advantages: Higher yield of viable SVF cells although this again can vary depending on equipment technology.

- Efficiency: More efficient and consistent separation process.

- Disadvantages: Potential for enzymatic contamination, although very minimal.

- Cost: Higher cost due to enzymes and additional regulatory requirements.

- Regulatory Challenges: Stricter regulations and approval processes due to the use of enzymes.

In summary, generally mechanical separation is safer, cost-effective, and easier to regulate, but typically yields fewer cells with potentially lower viability although it is also debated what higher viability actually is. Enzymatic separation yields a higher number of viable cells and is more efficient, but it involves higher costs, potential contamination, and stricter regulatory scrutiny.

Choosing the appropriate method depends on the specific clinical or research needs, considering factors like yield, cell viability, cost, and regulatory environment.

Culture and Expansion of SVF-Derived MSCs

This process is most often outsourced to personal stem cell banking service labs although it can also be done in-house.

Seeding and Culture: The isolated SVF cells are seeded in culture flasks and maintained in a suitable culture medium, often supplemented with fetal bovine serum (FBS) and growth factors.

Expansion: MSCs within the SVF adhere to the plastic surface of the culture flask and start to proliferate. Non-adherent cells are removed during media changes. The MSCs are expanded until they reach the desired confluence, usually 70-80%.

Characterization: The expanded MSCs are characterized by their morphology, growth rate, and the expression of specific surface markers (e.g., CD73, CD90, CD105) to confirm their mesenchymal stem cell identity.

We know little about the differences of these MSC sources. (SVF)-derived mesenchymal stem cells (MSCs) exhibit different CD markers compared to other sources of MSCs, such as those derived from bone marrow or umbilical cord tissue. Here are some key differences:

- SVF-derived MSCs typically express common MSC markers such as: CD73, CD90, CD105

- Absence of Hematopoietic Markers: Like other MSCs, SVF-derived MSCs lack hematopoietic markers, such as: CD34, CD45

- Additional Markers Specific to SVF-derived MSCs: Some unique markers often found in SVF-derived MSCs include: CD10, CD13, CD36, CD44

These markers help distinguish SVF-derived MSCs from other MSCs and indicate their origin from adipose tissue. Understanding these differences is important for their application in regenerative medicine and tissue engineering.

CD Marker	Umbilical Cord MSCs	Bone Marrow MSCs	SVF-Derived MSCs
CD73	Present	Present	Present
CD90	Present	Present	Present
CD105	Present	Present	Present
CD34	Absent	Absent	Variable
CD45	Absent	Absent	Absent
CD10	Absent	Absent	Present
CD13	Absent	Absent	Present
CD36	Absent	Absent	Present
CD44	Present	Present	Present
HLA-DR	Absent	Absent	Absent

Major Cytokine Differences

Cytokine	Umbilical Cord MSCs	Bone Marrow MSCs	SVF-Derived MSCs
IL-6	High	Moderate	High
IL-8	Moderate	High	High
TGF-β	High	High	High
VEGF	High	High	High
TNF-α	Low	Low	Low

Table 3: Comparative overview, highlighting the unique characteristics of MSCs derived from different tissues. Understanding these differences is crucial for optimizing their therapeutic applications.

Notes: CD markers help identify and differentiate MSCs from various sources. While common MSC markers such as CD73, CD90, and CD105 are present across all sources, specific markers like CD10, CD13, and CD36 are more prominent in SVF-derived MSCs.

Cytokine Profiles: Cytokine production varies among MSC sources, influencing their immunomodulatory and regenerative properties. For example, umbilical cord MSCs often produce higher levels of IL-6 and TGF-β compared to other sources.

Utilization of SVF-Derived MSCs

Harvesting and Preparation: Once the MSCs are expanded to the required number, they are harvested and prepared for therapeutic use. Depending on the application, they may be concentrated or mixed with other components.

Administration: SVF-derived MSCs can be administered directly into the target tissue or via intravenous infusion, depending on the intended therapeutic application, such as tissue repair, anti-inflammatory treatments, or cosmetic procedures.

Follow-Up: Patients are monitored for any adverse reactions post-treatment and followed up to assess the efficacy of the therapy in terms of symptom relief, tissue regeneration, and functional improvement.

The use of SVF-derived MSCs from adipose tissue offers a minimally invasive and abundant source of stem cells for regenerative medicine. The isolation, culture, and application of these cells require careful techniques to ensure their safety and efficacy in therapeutic settings.

Mesenchymal stem cells (MSCs) isolated from Umbilical cord.

Umbilical Cord Tissue Offers the Greatest Number of Harvestable Mesenchymal Stem Cells for Research and Clinical Application.

Vangsness 2015: "Yields for adipose tissue ranged from 4,737 cells/mL of tissue to 1,550,000 cells/mL of tissue. Yields for bone marrow ranged from 1 to 30 cells/mL to 317,400 cells/mL. Yields for umbilical cord tissue ranged from 10,000 cells/mL to 4,700,000 cells/cm of umbilical cord." Although these numbers can greatly vary with techniques and sources. [PMID26354202]

Mesenchymal stem cells (MSCs) isolated from Wharton's jelly of the umbilical cord are a promising source for regenerative medicine due to their high proliferation rate, immunomodulatory properties, and potential for differentiation. Here's an overview of the techniques used to isolate MSCs from Wharton's jelly:

Collection and Preparation

Umbilical Cord Collection: The umbilical cord is obtained after childbirth, with proper consent and following ethical guidelines. It is typically collected in a sterile container and transported to the laboratory for processing.

Dissection: The umbilical cord is washed with a sterile saline solution to remove blood and debris. The cord is then cut into segments, and the blood vessels (two arteries and one vein) are carefully removed to expose Wharton's jelly.

Isolation of MSCs - Enzymatic Digestion: Wharton's jelly is subjected to enzymatic digestion using collagenase and/or hyaluronidase to release the MSCs. The digestion is carried out at 37°C for a specific duration, usually a few hours.

Mechanical Method: Alternatively, a mechanical method can be used, where Wharton's jelly is minced into small pieces and then gently agitated to release the cells without the use of enzymes.

Centrifugation: After digestion or mechanical processing, the cell suspension is centrifuged to separate the MSCs from the digested tissue and enzymes.

Washing and Seeding: The cell pellet is washed with a phosphate-buffered saline (PBS) solution and then resuspended in a suitable culture medium. The cells are seeded in culture flasks and incubated at 37°C in a humidified atmosphere with 5% CO_2.

Culture and Expansion

Adherence and Expansion: MSCs from Wharton's jelly will adhere to the plastic surface of the culture flask. After 24-48 hours, non-adherent cells are removed by changing the medium. The adherent MSCs are allowed to proliferate until they reach 70-80% confluence.

Passaging: Once the MSCs reach the desired confluence, they are detached using trypsin-EDTA, counted, and subcultured (passaged) into new flasks for further expansion.

Characterization: The isolated MSCs are characterized based on their morphology, surface marker expression (e.g., CD73, CD90, CD105), and differentiation potential into osteocytes, chondrocytes, and adipocytes.

The isolation of MSCs from Wharton's jelly involves a combination of enzymatic digestion or mechanical processing, followed by culture and expansion in vitro. These techniques allow for the procurement of a significant number of MSCs, which can be used for various applications in regenerative medicine and research. In addition many more birth tissues are included here such as the cord blood itself, placental tissue and amniotic fluid.

Do Umbilical MSCs transfer foreign DNA?

Allogeneic stem cell transplants using umbilical cord-derived stem cells, such as mesenchymal stem cells (MSCs), are primarily used for their regenerative, immunomodulatory, and anti-inflammatory properties. Allogeneic mesenchymal stem cells (MSCs) from sources like umbilical cord tissue typically do not engraft or permanently integrate into the recipient's tissues. Instead, they exert their therapeutic effects through several mechanisms that do not involve long-term implantation or incorporation into the host tissue. Here's how they work:

Mechanisms of Action

These transplants do not involve the transfer of DNA or the integration of donor DNA into the recipient's genome. Only a short term presence of the donor's DNA is evident and no long-term engraftment has been found to our current knowledge.

Short-Term Persistence: Some studies have reported the transient presence of donor cell DNA in recipients after allogeneic MSC transplantation. However, this presence is usually short-lived and does not indicate long-term engraftment or integration into the host genome. We know from tissue culture experiments that UC-MSCs can only undergo a finite number of population doublings before they enter a state of senescence. The number of population doublings varies depending on the specific cell isolate and culture conditions. [PMID18493317]

Limited Engraftment: There is limited evidence of actual engraftment of allogeneic MSCs into host tissues. When detected, the engraftment is usually at very low levels and may not have functional significance.

Clinical Implications: The potential clinical implications of detecting donor DNA in recipients are not fully understood and are an area of ongoing research. The transient presence of donor DNA is generally not considered to pose a significant risk in the context of MSC therapies.

Sensitivity of Detection Methods: The ability to detect donor DNA depends on the sensitivity of the detection methods used. More sensitive techniques may detect low levels of donor DNA that are not clinically significant.

Route of Administration: The route of MSC administration (e.g., intravenous, intra-articular) may influence the likelihood of detecting donor DNA in different tissues.

Time of Sampling: The presence of donor DNA may vary over time, with a higher likelihood of detection shortly after transplantation and a decrease over time as the cells are cleared from the recipient's body.

Allogeneic MSCs are Not 'Gene Therapy'

To summarize the differences to genetically altered cells it is important once again to characterize MSCs:

Transient Presence: Allogeneic MSCs from the umbilical cord are typically transiently present in the recipient's body. They exert their therapeutic effects and are eventually cleared without engrafting or transferring their DNA to the recipient's cells.

No Gene Integration: Unlike gene therapy, which involves the deliberate modification of the recipient's genetic material with genetically modified vectors such as viruses, allogeneic stem cell transplants do not *aim* to alter the recipient's DNA.

Regulatory agencies, such as the FDA, distinguish between stem cell therapies and gene therapies based on their mechanism of action. Allogeneic umbilical cord stem cell transplants are classified as biological cell therapies, not gene therapies.

A new scientific focus involves Mitochondrial DNA transfer from MSCs to other cells. It is an emerging area of research with potential implications for understanding cellular communication, rescuing mitochondrial dysfunction, and developing regenerative therapies and cancer. Further studies are needed to elucidate the mechanisms, functional consequences, and therapeutic potential of mtDNA transfer in various disease contexts. [PMID33365311]

In conclusion, while there is some evidence of the transient presence of donor DNA in recipients after allogeneic MSC transplantation, this does not necessarily indicate long-term engraftment or functional integration. The detection of donor DNA is generally considered to be of limited clinical significance in the context of MSC therapies. Further research is needed to fully understand the implications of donor DNA presence and its relevance to the safety and efficacy of allogeneic stem cell treatments. Allogeneic umbilical cord stem cell transplants are used for their regenerative and immunomodulatory properties, not for transferring DNA or altering the recipient's genetic makeup. They are distinct from gene therapy and are primarily aimed at promoting tissue repair and modulating immune responses without integrating into the recipient's genome.

The Paracrine Mechanisms of Action

What do MSCs actually do if they are not acting on the DNA level? It is proposed that MSCs work by the following proposed mechanisms which will be discussed in more detail later.

Paracrine Signaling:

MSCs secrete a range of bioactive molecules, including growth factors, cytokines, and exosomes, which can modulate the local tissue environment, reduce inflammation, and promote healing and regeneration.

Immunomodulation:

These cells can modulate the immune response by interacting with various immune cells, potentially reducing autoimmune reactions and promoting a more regenerative environment.

Trophic Support:

MSCs provide trophic support to the damaged tissue by secreting factors that enhance cell survival, proliferation, and differentiation.

In summary, MSCs exert their therapeutic effects through several mechanisms that do not involve long-term implantation or incorporation into the host tissue. Instead MSCs rather work as directors of an orchestra within the body.

Inflammation

Immunomodulation and the effect on inflammation is likely the first step in MSC action. This will be discussed in more detail and in the context of omega-3. In order to elaborate on the anti-inflammatory action of MSCs we dive right into a few clinical examples. Let us first talk about a few important inflammatory medical conditions where the effects of immune modulation are important. Although everyone wants to know if stem cells can help their particular medical condition, diving deeper into details of each condition would be far beyond the scope of this book. You will find a large selection of conditions here: https://omega3health.us/regenerative.

Here are just a few recent studies showing how MSCs exert their anti-inflammatory effects on various inflammatory disease conditions:

1. PCOS (Polycystic Ovary Syndrome) has a strong inflammatory component that can be modulated by MSCs. Nejabati 2024: Therapeutic Potential of Mesenchymal Stem Cells in PCOS: "Some research also indicates that umbilical cord mesenchymal stem cells (UC-MSCs) alleviate the inflammation of granulosa cells in women with PCOS." This review summarizes the current knowledge on the therapeutic potential of three types of MSCs: BMMSCs, AdMSCs, UC-MSCs and their secretome in the treatment of PCOS. In particular umbilical cord mesenchymal stem cells (UC-MSCs) alleviate the inflammation of granulosa cells in women with PCOS. [PMID37198984]

Chugh 2021: Our results suggest that BM-hMSC can reverse PCOS-induced inflammation through IL-10 secretion. BM-hMSC might be a novel and robust therapeutic approach for PCOS treatment. The anti-inflammatory cytokine interleukin-10 (IL-10) played a key role in mediating the effects of BM-hMSC and restored reproductive markers and fertility. [PMID34233746]

2. Multiple sclerosis (MS) is a chronic, neuroinflammatory, and demyelinating disease of the central nervous system (CNS). Jafarinia 2023: "Recent studies suggest that MSCs exert their effects through extracellular vesicles (EVs) released from the cells, rather than direct cellular engraftment or differentiation. This discovery has sparked interest in the potential of MSC-derived EVs as a cell-free therapy for MS. The mechanisms involved immunomodulation through effects on T cells, cytokines, CNS inflammation, and demyelination. " MSC-EVs from various tissue sources, such as bone marrow, adipose tissue, and umbilical cord, were found to reduce clinical scores and slow down disease progression! [PMID38163474]

3. Organ Transplants: The topic of *Graft-Versus-Host Disease* (GVHD) is discussed extensively in Part I and II. The immunomodulatory functions of human MSCs are now being used to alleviate organ rejections. Miura 2013: "Multipotent mesenchymal stem/stromal cells (MSCs) have been extensively used as a transplantable cell source for regenerative medicine and immunomodulatory therapy. Specifically in allogeneic hematopoietic stem cell transplantation (HSCT), co-transplantation or post-transplant infusion of MSCs derived from bone marrow (BM) of non-self donors has been implicated in accelerating hematopoietic recovery, ameliorating Graft-Versus-Host Disease, and promoting tissue regeneration." Addressing these concerns, hydrogel encapsulation emerges as a promising solution to enhance the therapeutic effectiveness of MSCs in vivo. [PMID38334602]

Aggarwal 2005 "We examined the immunomodulatory functions of human MSCs (hMSCs) by co-culturing them with purified subpopulations of immune cells and report here that hMSCs altered the cytokine secretion profile of dendritic cells (DCs), naive and effector T cells (T helper 1 [T(H)1] and T(H)2), and natural killer (NK) cells to induce a more anti-inflammatory or tolerant phenotype." The data may offer insights into the interactions between allogeneic MSCs and immune cells and provide mechanisms likely involved with the in vivo MSC-mediated induction of tolerance that could be therapeutic for reduction of GVHD. [PMID15494428]

4. Liver Disease: Chronic liver disease can result from various causes such as hepatitis infections (Hepatitis B and C), alcohol-related liver disease, non-alcoholic fatty liver disease (NAFLD), and autoimmune liver diseases. Each type has its own progression pattern and potential outcomes. Over time, chronic liver disease can lead to complications such as cirrhosis (scarring of the liver), which can severely impair liver function. Advanced cirrhosis may lead to liver failure, a life-threatening condition that might require a liver transplant. Zhu 2024: "The elucidation of the role of MSC-EVs in the recovery and repair of hepatic tissues, as well as their contribution to maintaining tissue homeostasis, is discussed in relation to different chronic liver diseases. This review aims to provide new insights into the unique roles that MSC-EVs play in the treatment of chronic liver diseases." According to research, MSC exosomes can maintain tissue homeostasis, which is necessary for healthy tissue function and elucidate the role of MSC-EVs in the recovery and repair of hepatic tissues! [PMID38223423]

"MSC-derived extracellular vesicles (MSC-EVs) can inhibit the activation and proliferation of a variety of proinflammatory cells, such as Th1, Th17 and M1 macrophages, reducing the secretion of proinflammatory cytokines, while promoting the proliferation of anti-inflammatory cells, such as M2 macrophages and Tregs, and increasing the secretion of anti-inflammatory cytokines, thus playing a role in immune regulation and exhibiting immunomodulatory functions. This article focuses on the immunomodulatory effects of MSC-EVs and summarizes the pivotal roles of MSC-EVs as a cell-free therapy in liver diseases, including NAFLD, AIH, acute liver failure, liver fibrosis and hepatic ischemia-reperfusion injury. [PMID35309311]

5. Alzheimer's disease and other neuro-degenerative diseases:

Alzheimer's disease (AD) is increasingly recognized not just as a neurodegenerative condition but also one involving significant inflammatory processes within the brain. This inflammation is believed to contribute to the progression of the disease by exacerbating neuronal damage. Mesenchymal stem cells (MSCs) have garnered attention as a potential therapeutic approach to manage or possibly alter the course of Alzheimer's due to their unique anti-inflammatory and regenerative capabilities. Here's an overview of how MSC therapy could impact Alzheimer's disease:

MSCs can modulate immune responses, potentially reducing chronic inflammation in the brain which is associated with Alzheimer's. They achieve this by secreting anti-inflammatory cytokines and by interacting with various immune cells, altering their function towards a more regulated state. [PMID32496649]

Neuroprotection: Beyond their immunomodulatory effects, MSCs may provide neuroprotective benefits. They can secrete growth factors that support neuronal survival and promote the repair of damaged neural tissue.

As a potential mechanism in Alzheimer's Disease some studies suggest that MSCs might influence the mechanisms involved in the clearance of amyloid-beta, a protein that accumulates abnormally in Alzheimer's and contributes to neuronal damage.

Tackling Tau Pathology: MSCs could potentially impact the pathology related to tau, another protein that forms harmful tangles in the brains of Alzheimer's patients.

Promoting Neurogenesis: There is evidence that MSC treatment might encourage neurogenesis (growth of new neurons) in the adult brain, which could help in replacing neurons lost to the degenerative processes of Alzheimer's. Ye 2024: "MSC-EVs participate in chronic inflammatory and immune processes by transferring nucleic acids, proteins and lipids from the parent cell to the recipient cell, thus MSC-EVs retain their immunomodulatory capacity while avoiding the safety issues associated with living cell therapy, making them a promising focus for immunomodulatory therapy." [PMID38259476]

6. Autoimmune Disease: Autoimmune diseases represent a broad category of conditions in which the immune system mistakenly attacks the body's own tissues, leading to chronic inflammation and various symptoms. These diseases can manifest in many forms, including rheumatoid arthritis (RA), Hashimoto's thyroiditis, lupus, and many others. Mesenchymal stem cells (MSCs) are being explored as a potential treatment for these conditions due to their immunomodulatory and anti-inflammatory properties. Here's how MSCs could play a role in managing autoimmune diseases:

MSCs have the ability to modulate immune responses by interacting with various immune cells such as T cells, B cells, dendritic cells, and macrophages. They can promote a shift from a pro-inflammatory environment to a more regulated or anti-inflammatory state.

MSCs secrete a range of bioactive molecules that can suppress inflammatory responses. These include cytokines such as TGF-β (transforming growth factor-beta) and IL-10 (interleukin-10), which help regulate immune cell functions.

Shen 2021: "Moreover, substantial progress has been made in the treatment of autoimmune diseases, including multiple sclerosis (MS), systemic lupus erythematosus (SLE), type-1 diabetes (T1DM), uveitis, rheumatoid arthritis (RA), and inflammatory bowel disease (IBD). [PMID34646275]

Huang 2022: "The secretome of MSCs consists of cytokines, chemokines, signaling molecules, and growth factors, which effectively contribute to the regulation of immune and inflammatory responses. The immunomodulatory effects of MSCs can also be achieved through direct cell contact with microenvironmental factors and immune cells. Furthermore, preconditioned and engineered MSCs can specifically improve the immunomodulation effects in diverse clinical applications. "[PMID36077421]

In summary, this very small but representative excerpt of recent publications shows the immune modulatory effects of MSCs. Much research has to be done to fully understand these mechanisms especially on a cellular level. For a deeper dive, we now have a look at cytokines and interleukins.

The Role of Interleukins - Umbilical MSCs

For a deeper dive, Let us specifically discuss the role of cytokines (small proteins that are controlling the growth and activity of cells part of immune system). Mesenchymal stem cells (MSCs) derived from umbilical cord tissue possess significant anti-inflammatory properties, primarily mediated through the release of various cytokines, including interleukins. These anti-inflammatory molecules play a vital role in modulating the immune response, which is particularly relevant in treating inflammatory and autoimmune diseases.

Key Interleukins and Markers:

- IL-10 (Interleukin-10): A pivotal anti-inflammatory cytokine that helps suppress inflammatory responses and promote tissue healing.

- TGF-β (Transforming Growth Factor-beta): Involved in tissue regeneration and immune regulation, TGF-β is crucial for its anti-inflammatory effects.

- PGE2 (Prostaglandin E2): Generally a pro-inflammatory eicosanoid, when secreted by MSCs PGE2 can modulate the immune system and suppresses inflammatory responses.

- PGE3 (Prostaglandin E3): The combined action of MSCs and PGE3 (anti-inflammatory) can lead to improved outcomes in tissue repair.

Proteomics of MSC Secretome and Umbilical Tissue: Recent reviews in proteomics have shed light on the complex composition of the MSC secretome and umbilical tissue. These studies reveal a diverse array of proteins, including growth factors, cytokines, and extracellular matrix proteins, which contribute to their therapeutic potential.

Nature's Anti-Inflammatory Message in Birth Tissue: The presence of anti-inflammatory compounds in birth tissues, such as the placenta and umbilical cord, is a fascinating aspect of human physiology. This natural anti-inflammatory environment is thought to play several critical roles:

Protecting the Fetus: It helps in protecting the fetus, which is a semi-allogeneic entity, from being attacked by the mother's immune system.

Facilitating Tolerance: These molecules promote immune tolerance, which is crucial during pregnancy and at the time of birth.

Aiding in the Birthing Process: The anti-inflammatory environment may help in reducing tissue damage and inflammation during childbirth, aiding in recovery post-delivery.

Implications for Regenerative Medicine:

Understanding the anti-inflammatory properties of umbilical MSCs opens up new avenues for treating a range of inflammatory and autoimmune disorders. By harnessing these properties, therapies can potentially reduce disease symptoms and facilitate tissue repair and regeneration.

Future Research and Clinical Applications: Ongoing research is focused on further unraveling the complex molecular mechanisms behind the anti-inflammatory effects of umbilical MSCs. This knowledge is crucial for developing targeted therapies that can effectively utilize these natural properties for clinical applications.

The exploration of anti-inflammatory markers, particularly interleukins in umbilical MSCs, offers significant insights into the therapeutic potential of these cells. The natural anti-inflammatory properties of birth tissues represent a unique aspect of human biology, with promising implications for regenerative medicine. As we continue to uncover the secrets of these remarkable cells, we move closer to developing more effective treatments for a wide range of inflammatory and autoimmune conditions.

The Dual Role of PGE2 in Immune Biochemistry and MSCs from Umbilical Tissue

The role of bioactive molecules like PGE2 (Prostaglandin E2) in immune responses and inflammation is not black and white. The complex interplay between promoting and resolving inflammation is a critical aspect of the body's response to injury and infection. Here's a more detailed nuanced view of how MSCs modulate inflammation.

Pro-inflammatory Phase:

Initially, in response to injury or infection, the body triggers an inflammatory response. PGE2, as a pro-inflammatory eicosanoid, plays a significant role in this phase. It helps in vasodilation (widening of blood vessels), increasing vascular permeability, and sensitizing nerve endings to pain, which are hallmarks of inflammation.

This response is crucial for combating pathogens, removing damaged cells, and setting the stage for tissue repair.

Resolution of Inflammation:

After the initial inflammatory response, the body needs to resolve this inflammation to prevent chronic inflammation and enable healing. As this is supposed to be the job of anti-inflammatory eicosanoids, PGE2, in the context of MSCs, can also play a role in resolving inflammation.

The resolution phase *involves a shift* in the types of eicosanoids and cytokines produced. The same molecule, PGE2, can facilitate this transition. It can start acting in a way that suppresses certain immune responses and promotes the healing process. [PMID36830980]

Context and Concentration-Dependent Effects: The effects of PGE2 are highly dependent on the context and its concentration in the tissue environment. In different concentrations and at different stages of the immune response, PGE2 can have varying effects.

Role in MSCs and Umbilical Tissue: In the specific context of MSCs, including those derived from umbilical cord tissue, PGE2 contributes to the immunomodulatory effects of these cells. Here, PGE2 can help skew the immune response towards a more anti-inflammatory or tolerant state, beneficial in controlling excessive or chronic inflammation.

Human UC-MSCs and Their Ability to Engulf Apoptotic Cells

Human umbilical cord-derived mesenchymal stem cells (UC-MSCs) have demonstrated a remarkable ability to engulf apoptotic cells, a process known as efferocytosis. This ability contributes significantly to their therapeutic potential in regenerative medicine and immune modulation.

Mechanism: UC-MSCs can recognize and engulf apoptotic cells through specific cell surface receptors. This process involves the binding of apoptotic cells to these receptors, followed by internalization and degradation.

Receptors Involved: Common receptors involved in efferocytosis include TAM receptors (Tyro3, Axl, and MerTK), as well as integrins and phosphatidylserine receptors.

Immunomodulatory Effects: By engulfing apoptotic cells, UC-MSCs can secrete anti-inflammatory cytokines such as IL-10 and TGF-β, which help in resolving inflammation and promoting tissue repair.

Reduction of Pro-Inflammatory Signals: Efferocytosis by UC-MSCs leads to a decrease in pro-inflammatory cytokines like TNF-α and IL-6, further aiding in the reduction of inflammation.

Promotion of Tissue Repair: Secretion of Growth Factors: Following the engulfment of apoptotic cells, UC-MSCs release growth factors that promote tissue regeneration and healing. These factors include VEGF (vascular endothelial growth factor) and HGF (hepatocyte growth factor).

Enhanced Healing: The clearance of apoptotic cells prevents secondary necrosis and the release of potentially harmful cellular contents, thereby enhancing the overall healing process.

Immune Regulation: Modulation of Immune Cells: UC-MSCs can modulate the activity of various immune cells, including macrophages and dendritic cells, through efferocytosis. This modulation helps in maintaining a balanced immune response and preventing excessive inflammation.

In summary, Human UC-MSCs possess the ability to engulf apoptotic cells, contributing to their anti-inflammatory, immunomodulatory, and tissue repair capabilities. This efferocytosis process plays a crucial role in their therapeutic potential, making UC-MSCs a valuable tool in regenerative medicine and the treatment of inflammatory conditions. Understanding and harnessing this ability can lead to more effective and targeted stem cell therapies. [PMID31248835]

Complexity in Immune Regulation:

This complexity in immune regulation underscores the need for a balanced approach in treating inflammatory conditions. Understanding the dual role of molecules like PGE2 is crucial in designing therapies that can effectively manage the inflammatory response without hindering tissue repair and regeneration.

Zafranskaya 2013 concluded: "These results have demonstrated that in patients with multiple sclerosis (MS), PGE2 is one of the possible factors of MSC immunosuppression. The interrelation between PGE2 concentrations and T cell proliferation suppression mediated by MSC may explain one of the immune mechanisms of cell therapy" [PMID23944654]

Zhang 2022: Our results further showed that MSC-derived prostaglandin E2 (PGE2) likely promoted nicotinic acetylcholine (ACh) synthesis and release... we reveal a previously unrecognized MSC-mediated mechanism of CAP activation as the means by which MSCs alleviate ARDS-like syndrome, providing insight into the clinical translation of MSCs or CAP-related strategies for the treatment of patients with ARDS. [PMID36064538]

The immune system's biochemistry, particularly the role of molecules like PGE2, illustrates the delicate balance between initiating and resolving inflammation. This balance is vital for effective immune responses, preventing chronic inflammation, and ensuring proper healing and tissue repair. In regenerative medicine, leveraging this understanding is key to developing therapies that harness the body's natural healing mechanisms while keeping inflammatory responses in check.

MSCs Suppress Inflammation

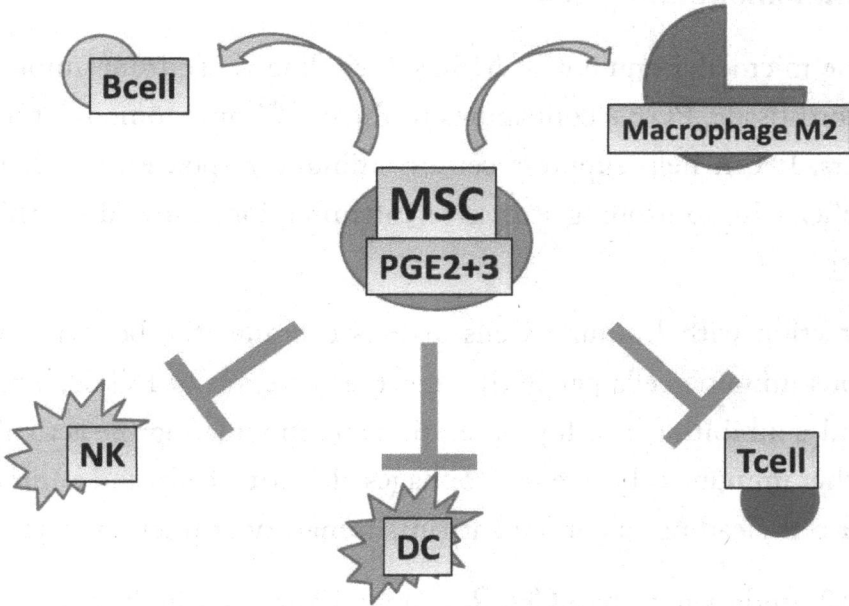

Fig.11: MSCs can modulate the inflammatory immune response of PGE2. They can inhibit the proliferation of T-cells, NK and dendritic cells contributing to an overall anti-inflammatory effect. The schematic illustrates these interactions, highlighting how MSCs and PGE2 influence different immune cells to create a balanced immune response. [PMID36830980]

How MSCs modulate PGE2

In the context of umbilical cord tissue and mesenchymal stem cells (MSCs) derived from this tissue, PGE2 can indeed exhibit anti-inflammatory properties, which is part of the unique and complex immunomodulatory functions of MSCs. This might seem counterintuitive given PGE2's general role in promoting inflammation, but in the environment of MSCs, the interactions and effects can be quite different.

Immunomodulatory Role:

In the microenvironment of MSCs, including those from umbilical cord tissue, PGE2 contributes to the cells' immunomodulatory effects. It can help suppress certain immune responses, which is beneficial in controlling excessive inflammation. How does this work?

Interaction with Immune Cells: MSCs can alter the behavior of various immune cells partly through the secretion of PGE2. This includes inhibiting T-cell proliferation and modulating the activity of other immune cells like macrophages, dendritic cells, and natural killer cells, leading to a more anti-inflammatory or tolerant state.

PGE2 Studies and Stem Cell Research: Several studies have investigated the immunomodulatory effects of MSCs, highlighting the role of PGE2 among other factors. Zhang 2019 "Human UC MSCs possessed the ability to engulf ACs. AC-MSCs increased MSC-mediated suppression of CD4+ T cell proliferation compared to MSCs alone. Mechanistically, ACs stimulated MSCs to express COX2 and consequently produced PGE2 that inhibited T cell responses." [PMID31248835]

Interaction of MSCs with PGE3

Mesenchymal stem cells (MSCs) interact with various prostaglandins, including Prostaglandin E3 (PGE3), which is derived from eicosapentaenoic acid (EPA), an omega-3 fatty acid as discussed later on. PGE3 has distinct anti-inflammatory properties compared to Prostaglandin E2 (PGE2), which is derived from arachidonic

154

acid (an omega-6 fatty acid). The interaction between MSCs and PGE3 plays a significant role in modulating the immune response and inflammation. [PMID18024478]

Anti-Inflammatory Properties of PGE3

- Reduction of Pro-Inflammatory Cytokines: PGE3 can decrease the production of pro-inflammatory cytokines such as TNF-α, IL-6, and IL-1β.

- Promotion of Anti-Inflammatory Cytokines: It can increase the production of anti-inflammatory cytokines like IL-10.

- Inhibition of NF-κB Pathway: PGE3 can inhibit the NF-κB signaling pathway, which is crucial for the expression of many pro-inflammatory genes.

MSCs and PGE3

- Enhanced Anti-Inflammatory Effects: MSCs can further enhance the anti-inflammatory effects of PGE3. By secreting bioactive molecules, MSCs modulate the immune response to create a more favorable environment for tissue repair and regeneration.

- Immunomodulation: MSCs, through their interaction with PGE3, can inhibit the proliferation of pro-inflammatory immune cells and promote the differentiation and activity of regulatory T cells (Tregs) and other anti-inflammatory immune cells.

- Promotion of Tissue Repair: The combined action of MSCs and PGE3 can lead to improved outcomes in tissue repair and regeneration by reducing chronic inflammation and promoting a more balanced immune response.

Mechanisms of Interaction

Receptor-Mediated Actions: MSCs express receptors (eg. PPAR) for prostaglandins, including those for PGE3. Through these receptors, MSCs can respond to PGE3 in their environment, adjusting their secretion profile of cytokines and growth factors. [PMID32651456]

Paracrine Signaling: MSCs and PGE3 work together in a paracrine manner, where PGE3 influences the MSCs' behavior, and MSCs secrete factors that further amplify the anti-inflammatory effects of PGE3.

The interaction between MSCs and PGE3 enhances the anti-inflammatory and immunomodulatory effects crucial for effective tissue repair and regeneration. This synergy helps in creating an environment conducive to healing by reducing chronic inflammation and promoting tissue homeostasis. Understanding these interactions is vital for developing MSC-based therapies for inflammatory and immune-related conditions. In this context it is important that the body has adequate amounts (>8%) of Omega-3. Unfortunately most Americans have less than 2.5% functional EPA and DHA in their cell membrane.

In conclusion, in the environment of MSCs, especially those derived from sources like the umbilical cord, the role of PGE2 is multifaceted. It can act in a unique anti-inflammatory manner, contributing to the therapeutic potential of MSCs in treating various inflammatory and autoimmune conditions. This illustrates the complex nature of biological signaling molecules, where the context and microenvironment significantly influence their effects.

What role does PGE2 play in bone healing?

Mesenchymal stem cell–macrophage crosstalk and bone healing:

The process of bone healing is a prime example of how the immune system and regenerative mechanisms work together, and it illustrates the complex interplay between different cell types and signaling molecules. [PMID29329642] Specifically, the roles of macrophages and their secreted molecules such as Oncostatin M, Prostaglandin E2 (PGE2), and Bone Morphogenetic Protein-2 (BMP2) are crucial in this process. Let's explore this in the context of the differentiation of mesenchymal stem cells (MSCs) along the osteogenic pathway.

The MSC Role of Macrophage Polarization in Fracture Healing

Here is an example of how specifically MSCs can assist in a healing process in the body:

Importance in Fracture Healing

- Transition: The shift from M1 to M2 macrophages is essential for transitioning from inflammation to tissue repair.

- Regeneration: Promotes bone regeneration, reduces chronic inflammation, and improves overall healing outcomes.

Clinical Implications

Therapies: Targeting macrophage polarization could enhance fracture healing, potentially involving treatments that promote M2 macrophage activity.

Understanding the role of MSCs in manipulating the balance between M1 and M2 macrophages offers potential therapeutic avenues for improving fracture healing and recovery.

The shift from M1 to M2 macrophages is essential for transitioning from inflammation to tissue repair and regeneration: The shift promotes bone regeneration, reduces chronic inflammation, and improves overall healing outcomes.

1. Initial Inflammatory Phase (M1 Dominance):

Following a bone fracture, the body's immediate response is inflammation, critical for clearing debris and hting potential infections. M1 macrophages, which are pro-inflammatory, dominate this phase, releasing cytokines and other factors that create an inflammatory "hot spot."

2. Transition to Soft Callus Formation (M2 Dominance):

As healing progresses, the inflammatory phase gives way to a regeneration phase. This is marked by the formation of a soft callus, a temporary structure that stabilizes the fracture. During this phase, M2 macrophages, known for their tissue healing and anti-inflammatory roles, become more prevalent. They secrete factors that promote tissue repair, angiogenesis (formation of new blood vessels), and eventually the mineralization of the soft callus into hard bone.

Macrophage-Derived Signaling in Bone Healing

The Healing Process involves the following phases over the time of several weeks and months.

- Inflammatory Phase: M1 macrophages help in cleaning the fracture site.

- Repair Phase: M2 macrophages support the formation of new tissues and blood vessels, crucial for effective healing.

- Remodeling Phase: M2 macrophages continue to facilitate tissue regeneration and remodeling.

1. Macrophage Polarization:

Macrophages can exhibit different phenotypes, primarily categorized as M1 (pro-inflammatory) and M2 (anti-inflammatory or tissue regenerative).

- M1 macrophages are associated with the early inflammatory response to injury, secreting cytokines and molecules that hit infection and clear damaged tissue.

- M2 macrophages are involved in the later stages of healing, promoting tissue repair and regeneration.

2. Role of Oncostatin M, PGE2, and BMP2:

- Oncostatin M: This cytokine, produced by macrophages, plays a role in bone remodeling and regeneration. It can influence MSCs and osteoblasts, aiding in bone repair.

- Prostaglandin E2 (PGE2): As previously discussed, PGE2 has dual roles. In bone healing, it can contribute both to the initial inflammatory response and later to the resolution and regeneration phase.

- Bone Morphogenetic Protein-2 (BMP2): BMP2 is a critical growth factor in bone formation, driving the differentiation of MSCs into osteoblasts, the cells responsible for bone formation.

3. Influence on MSC Differentiation:

- The differentiation of MSCs into osteoblasts (bone-forming cells) is a key step in bone healing. The microenvironment, enriched with cytokines and growth factors from macrophages, guides this process.

- The balance between M1 and M2 macrophages, and the timing of their respective signaling molecule secretions, influences how effectively MSCs differentiate and contribute to bone healing.

Current Understanding of macrophage interaction

1. Complex Interactions: The interplay between M1 and M2 macrophages, and their impact on MSC differentiation, is complex. While M1 macrophages initiate the inflammatory response, M2 macrophages promote healing. The sequential activation and interaction of these macrophage types are crucial for successful bone regeneration.

2. Relative Importance in MSC Differentiation: The exact roles and relative importance of M1 and M2 macrophages in guiding MSC differentiation towards the osteogenic pathway are still not fully understood. Research is ongoing to decipher these intricate mechanisms.

3. Future Research Directions: Much research is needed to understand the precise signaling pathways and interactions between macrophages, MSCs, and other cells involved in bone healing. Such

knowledge could lead to targeted therapies that enhance bone repair, such as in cases of fractures or osteoporosis.

For bone healing to occur, the orchestrated actions of macrophages and their signaling molecules play a pivotal role in guiding MSC differentiation and subsequent bone regeneration. Understanding the nuanced roles of different macrophage phenotypes and their interactions with MSCs is key to unlocking new potential in regenerative medicine, particularly for conditions related to bone health and repair. [PMID29329642]

Zhao 2022: "Macrophages and Bone Marrow-Derived Mesenchymal Stem Cells Work in Concert to Promote Fracture Healing" [PMID35196145]

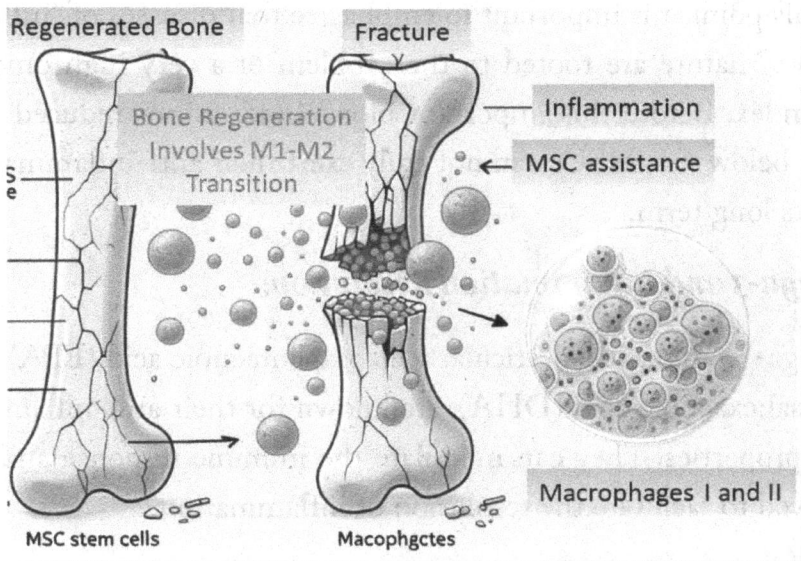

Fig.12: MSCs were shown to assist in macrophage crosstalk and the bone healing process. Specifically they assist the switch from M1 to M2 macrophages. [PMID29329642]

In summary, the healing process of a bone fracture is a highly orchestrated series of events that involve both inflammatory and regenerative phases. The transition from an initial inflammatory phase, predominantly mediated by M1 macrophages, to a tissue regeneration phase, largely facilitated by M2 macrophages, is crucial for effective healing. This transition is marked by the formation of a soft callus around the fracture site, which is a key step in the bone healing process. The role of omega-3 fatty acids in this transition together with MSCs is also an area of growing interest.

Omega-3 Fatty Acids assist MSCs

At this point it is important to emphasize that diseases of "inflammatory" nature are rooted to the problem of a very high omega-6/3 index. Before this important blood index is not reduced to a value below 4:1, MSCs can not truly exert their anti-inflammatory effects long term.

Omega-3 and Inflammation Resolution:

Omega-3 fatty acids, particularly eicosapentaenoic acid (EPA) and docosahexaenoic acid (DHA), are known for their anti-inflammatory properties. They can modulate the immune response and are believed to facilitate the resolution of inflammation.

1. Influencing Macrophage Polarization: Research suggests that omega-3 fatty acids can influence macrophage polarization, promoting the transition from the M1 to the M2 phenotype. This could be crucial in shifting the healing process from inflammation to regeneration.

2. Impact on Bone Healing: Omega-3 fatty acids may play a role in enhancing bone healing. By supporting the shift to M2 macrophages and reducing prolonged inflammation, they potentially contribute to the formation and mineralization of the callus.

3. Dietary and Supplemental Implications: This understanding underscores the potential importance of diet and supplementation in bone health and healing. Adequate intake of omega-3 fatty acids, through diet or supplements, could be beneficial in the context of bone fracture healing.

While the beneficial effects of omega-3 fatty acids on general inflammation are well-recognized, their specific role in bone healing and macrophage polarization is an area of active research. Future studies are needed to fully elucidate these mechanisms and to translate this knowledge into clinical practice.

The shift from an M1-dominated inflammatory response to an M2-dominated regenerative phase is a critical aspect of bone healing. Omega-3 fatty acids may play a significant role in this transition, potentially enhancing the healing process. This insight opens up possibilities for nutritional and therapeutic strategies to support bone health and recovery from fractures.

In summary, both Omega3 and MSCs integrate each other's role in the immunomodulation of ECM as well as cytokine components. Casado-Diaz 2013: "An increase in the intake of omega-3 respect to omega-6 may provide protection against the loss of bone mass, since omega-6 favors the osteoclastic activity by diminishing the opg/rankl gene expression in osteoblasts **and promotes MSC differentiation into adipocytes,** thus diminishing the production of osteoblasts." [PMID23104199]

Specialized Pro-Resolving Mediators - the answer to chronic inflammation

Omega-3 fatty acids plays a crucial role in the resolution of inflammation

Specialized Pro-Resolving Mediators (SPMs) are a group of bioactive lipid molecules derived from omega-3 fatty acids, such as eicosapentaenoic acid (EPA) and docosahexaenoic acid (DHA). These molecules play a crucial role in the resolution phase of inflammation, helping to terminate and resolve inflammatory responses and promote tissue healing. Recent research has also explored the interactions between SPMs and stem cells, particularly in the context of regenerative medicine.

Types of SPMs [PMID29757195]:

SPMs are produced by Omega3 species and include several families of molecules, such as lipoxins, resolvins, protectins, and maresins, each derived from different precursors within the omega-3 fatty acid pathway.

Anti-Inflammatory and Pro-Resolving Actions: Unlike traditional anti-inflammatory drugs that suppress inflammation, SPMs actively promote the resolution of inflammation. They do this by inhibiting the recruitment of additional immune cells to the site of inflammation and by stimulating the clearance of inflammatory cells and debris.

Tissue Protection and Healing: SPMs also promote tissue regeneration and healing by enhancing the repair of damaged tissues and by protecting tissues from further injury.

Modulation of Stem Cell Behavior:

SPMs can influence the behavior of stem cells, including mesenchymal stem cells (MSCs). They may enhance stem cell proliferation, migration, and differentiation, which are critical for tissue repair and regeneration.

Enhancement of Regenerative Therapies: Incorporating SPMs into regenerative therapies, such as stem cell transplantation, may enhance the efficacy of these treatments by reducing inflammation and promoting tissue healing.

SPM - Potential in Tissue Engineering:

SPMs have potential applications in tissue engineering, where they could be used to create a pro-resolving and regenerative microenvironment that supports the integration and function of engineered tissues.

Specialized Pro-Resolving Mediators derived from omega-3 fatty acids represent an important class of molecules that actively promote the resolution of inflammation and tissue healing. Their interactions with stem cells offer promising avenues for enhancing regenerative medicine and tissue engineering strategies. Much research is needed to fully understand the mechanisms of action of SPMs and their potential clinical applications in stem cell therapies.

In this context, testing the omega-3 index of the membranes is crucial! Proper supplementation with non-rancid omega-3 is needed to increase the omega-3 membrane amount to over 8%. Millions of tests show that the average person is 70% - 90% deficient with an index of less than 3%. This results in an inflammatory ratio of omega-6/3 of over 20:1 worldwide. This process of reducing your inflammatory index below 3:1 may take up to 3 years.

Reduction of Scar tissue: The Role of microRNAs in Umbilical MSCs

Exosomes and other cell-free MSC products

Exosomes and secretomes are discussed in further detail below. Essentially the paracrine effects of Mesenchymal Stem Cell (MSC) exosomes play a pivotal role in the regenerative and healing processes associated with MSC therapies. Exosomes are small extracellular vesicles released by cells, including MSCs, and they serve as carriers for various bioactive molecules such as proteins, lipids, mRNA, and microRNA. These exosomes act through a paracrine mechanism, meaning they exert their effects on nearby cells in the local tissue environment. Exosomes from MSCs can deliver a variety of RNA, proteins and lipids, thereby facilitating MSC migration and cartilage repair. [PMID37937669]

Here are a few examples of miRNAs that have been identified in MSC exosomes:

- miR-21: This miRNA is known to be involved in cell proliferation, apoptosis, and differentiation. MSC-derived exosomes containing miR-21 have been shown to promote angiogenesis and reduce fibrosis in a mouse model of myocardial infarction. (Source: Zhang et al., 2015)

- miR-146a: This miRNA is known to be involved in the regulation of immune responses and inflammation. MSC-derived exosomes containing miR-146a have been shown to attenuate inflammation and promote tissue regeneration in models of acute lung injury and liver fibrosis. (Source: Lou et al., 2020)

- miR-133a: This miRNA is known to be involved in muscle differentiation and regeneration. MSC-derived exosomes containing miR-133a have been shown to promote myogenesis and improve muscle function in a mouse model of muscular dystrophy. (Source: Yin et al., 2019)

- miR-122: This miRNA is highly expressed in liver tissue and is involved in the regulation of lipid metabolism. MSC-derived exosomes containing miR-122 have been shown to reduce hepatic steatosis and improve insulin sensitivity in a mouse model of nonalcoholic fatty liver disease. (Source: Liang et al., 2020)

Key Aspects of the Paracrine Effect of MSC Exosomes

Cell Communication and Signaling: MSC exosomes facilitate intercellular communication by transferring their cargo to target cells. This transfer can modulate cellular behaviors and responses in the recipient cells, influencing processes like inflammation, immune response, and tissue repair.

Modulation of Immune Responses: Exosomes can play a significant role in modulating the immune system. They carry anti-inflammatory and immunosuppressive molecules that can alter the behavior of various immune cells, thus contributing to the immunomodulatory effects of MSCs.

Promotion of Tissue Repair and Regeneration: MSC exosomes contain growth factors, cytokines, and other regenerative molecules that can stimulate tissue repair processes. They can enhance cell proliferation, angiogenesis (formation of new blood vessels), and the regeneration of damaged tissues.

Involvement in Wound Healing: In wound healing, exosomes from MSCs can accelerate the process by enhancing collagen synthesis, promoting angiogenesis, and reducing inflammation. [PMID37867186]

Impact on Tumor Microenvironment: There is emerging evidence that MSC exosomes can influence the tumor microenvironment, although this area is complex and requires further research to understand its implications fully.

Role in Neuroprotection: In neurodegenerative diseases, MSC exosomes have shown potential in providing neuroprotection and aiding in the repair of neural tissue, although the mechanisms and efficacy are still being explored.

Research and Clinical Implications: The understanding of MSC exosome-mediated paracrine effects is still evolving, with ongoing research aimed at unraveling the specific mechanisms and potential therapeutic applications.

Clinical applications of MSC exosomes are being explored in various fields, including regenerative medicine, immunotherapy, and tissue engineering including the use of new technologies like hydrogels. [PMID33445616]

Zhao 2023 "Engineering exosomes derived from subcutaneous fat MSCs specially promote cartilage repair as miR-199a-3p delivery vehicles in Osteoarthritis. Intra-articular injection of antagomiR-199a-3p dramatically attenuated the protective

effect of MSCsSC-Exos-mediated on articular cartilage in vivo."
[PMID37736726]

In summary, the paracrine effect of MSC exosomes represents a significant mechanism through which MSCs exert their therapeutic actions. These exosomes act as mediators in cell signaling and play a crucial role in modulating immune responses, promoting tissue repair, and influencing various physiological and pathological processes. As research in this area advances, the potential for utilizing MSC exosomes and their message in therapeutic applications continues to grow.

The 'Homing-in' Mechanisms

MSCs have a homing ability, meaning that they can migrate into injured sites, and they possess the capacity to differentiate into local components of injured sites and the ability to secrete chemokines, cytokines, and growth factors that help in tissue regeneration [PMID27010148]. Exosomes, which are small extracellular vesicles released by MSC cells, play a crucial role in cell-to-cell communication and can have significant effects on the behavior of recipient cells. One of the key features of exosomes is their ability to home to specific tissues and influence them through what is often described as a paracrine effect. Here's an overview of how exosome homing works and its implications:

Mechanisms of Exosome Homing

Targeted Delivery: Exosomes display specific surface proteins that can interact with receptors on target cells or tissues. This interaction facilitates the targeted delivery of exosomes to specific sites within the body.

Tissue-Specific Markers: The content and surface markers of exosomes often reflect their cell of origin and can influence their targeting behavior. Cells may modify exosomal content to specifically target certain tissues that express complementary receptors.

Microenvironmental Influences: The local microenvironment can influence exosome uptake. Factors such as pH, extracellular matrix components, and local enzyme activity can affect the stability and bioavailability of exosomes, thereby modulating their homing capabilities.

Fu 2019: "The migration of BMSCs is regulated by mechanical and chemical factors in this trafficking process. In this paper, we review the effects of several main regulatory factors on BMSC migration and its underlying mechanism; discuss two critical roles of BMSCs-namely, directed differentiation and the paracrine function-in tissue repair; and provide insight into the relationship between BMSC migration and tissue repair." [PMID31357692]

Chamberlain 2027: "Several studies have reported the functional expression of various chemokine receptors and adhesion molecules on human MSCs. Harnessing the migratory potential of MSCs by modulating their chemokine-chemokine receptor interactions may be a powerful way to increase their ability to correct inherited disorders of mesenchymal tissues or facilitate tissue repair in vivo." [PMID17656645]

Sterilized Secretome Products and Placental Derived Protein Array (PDPA)

As discussed in various chapters before cell-free "secretome products" may be the most promising future of "stem cell" therapy.

Sterilized Secretome Products from MSCs:

Definition: The secretome comprises the array of proteins, growth factors, cytokines, and extracellular vesicles (including exosomes) secreted by MSCs in culture.

Preparation: After MSCs are cultured, the conditioned medium containing the secretome is collected, concentrated, and sterilized to ensure safety for therapeutic use.

Applications: These products are used for their regenerative, anti-inflammatory, and immunomodulatory properties in conditions such as wound healing, osteoarthritis, and autoimmune diseases.

Advantages: Reduced risk of immune rejection compared to live cell therapies, standardized product consistency, and potential for use in allogeneic settings.

Placental Derived Protein Array (PDPA):

Another level of "cell free products" are Placental Derived Protein Array (PDPA). The term "Placental Derived Protein Array (PDPA)" does not yet refer to a widely recognized or standard technique or tool in the biomedical sciences. However, the term as it stands suggests a focus on proteins derived from placental tissue, possibly arrayed for the purpose of study or analysis. [PMID35773701] Given this interpretation, here's how a concept like PDPA can be understood or applied:

Definition: PDPA consists of proteins and growth factors derived from placental tissues, which are known for their rich content of bioactive molecules.

Source: These products are obtained from the placenta, specifically from amniotic membrane, chorionic villi, and Wharton's jelly, which are processed to extract the desired proteins.

Applications: Similar to MSC secretome, PDPA is used for its regenerative and anti-inflammatory effects, with applications in wound healing, tissue regeneration, and anti-aging treatments.

Advantages: High concentration of growth factors and cytokines, availability from a readily accessible source, and lower risk of disease transmission if properly processed.

Content: Both contain growth factors, cytokines, and extracellular vesicles, but MSC secretome is tailored to the cells' secretion profile, while PDPA is derived from a broader range of placental tissues.

Safety and Sterilization: Both require rigorous processing to ensure sterility and safety. MSC secretome products often undergo filtration and sterilization processes, while PDPA requires careful extraction and processing to maintain bioactivity.

Immunogenicity: MSC secretome products generally have low immunogenicity, making them suitable for allogeneic use. PDPA products, depending on the processing, can also have low immunogenicity but require thorough testing.

Efficacy: Both have shown promise in regenerative medicine, though direct comparisons in clinical efficacy are limited and depend on the specific application and formulation used.

PDPA- Placental Proteins:

The placenta is a rich source of various bioactive proteins and peptides that play crucial roles during pregnancy, including immune modulation, growth promotion, and tissue remodeling. These proteins might be of interest for various therapeutic and research purposes.

Protein Array: A protein array is a platform where a multitude of proteins are immobilized on a solid surface and used for high-throughput analysis, such as antibody binding studies, protein-protein interactions, or biomarker discovery.

Potential Applications of PDPA- Biomarker Research: Proteins derived from the placenta could be arrayed and analyzed to identify biomarkers of pregnancy-related disorders, such as pre-eclampsia, gestational diabetes, or preterm labor.

Drug Discovery: Identifying and characterizing placental proteins may help in discovering new drugs that could mimic or modulate the biological activities of these proteins, potentially leading to new treatments for a variety of conditions.

Therapeutic Proteins: New clinical data suggest that these PDPA samples are very powerful and are delivering clinical results quickly even in a lyophilised form. Some placental proteins have therapeutic potential due to their roles in immune modulation or tissue repair. A PDPA could facilitate the screening and analysis of these proteins for medical applications.

Research and Development

Developing a PDPA would involve isolating proteins from placental tissue, characterizing them, and effectively immobilizing them on an array. This requires advanced techniques in protein chemistry, surface chemistry, and possibly bioinformatics for data analysis.

Ethical Considerations: The use of PDPA as derived from human placental material, like any human-derived biological material, still involves ethical considerations regarding consent, potential risks, and the intended use of the derived data or products.

In summary, while the term "Placental Derived Protein Array (PDPA)" is not specifically recognized, the concept it suggests involves using advanced protein array technologies to study proteins derived from the placenta. This could have significant implications for medical research, particularly in understanding and treating pregnancy-related conditions. If you are referring to a specific product or research tool that has been developed recently or is known by this name in certain circles, further details from those specific contexts would be necessary to provide a more accurate and detailed explanation.

Summary:

Sterilized secretome products from MSC tissue cultures and PDPA both offer significant therapeutic potential, leveraging the regenerative and anti-inflammatory properties of their bioactive components. The choice between them depends on the specific clinical context, source availability, and desired therapeutic outcomes. Further research and clinical trials are essential to optimize their use and maximize their benefits in regenerative medicine.

Name of microRNA	General Gene Function	Wharton's Jelly	Amnion	Bone Marrow	Adipose	PRP
miR-21	Anti-apoptotic, proliferation	Yes	Yes	Yes	Yes	Yes
miR-145	Regulates cell differentiation	Yes	Yes	Yes	Yes	No
miR-155	Immune response modulator	Yes	Yes	Yes	Yes	Yes
miR-221	Cell cycle regulation	Yes	No	Yes	Yes	No
miR-140	Cartilage development, anti-inflammatory	Yes	Yes	No	No	No

Table 4: microRNA presence in MSC-rich tissues. These miRNAs are based on their general detection in studies focusing on miRNA profiles within these tissues. Actual miRNA content can vary based on specific conditions, extraction methods, and individual variability. For accurate and specific miRNA profiles, detailed molecular analyses such as quantitative PCR, miRNA sequencing, or miRNA microarray should be conducted on samples derived from these tissues. PRP (=platelet rich plasma); [PMID27252357, PMID29986939, PMID24268069, PMID36896010, PMID20668554].

MicroRNAs in Exosomes

MicroRNAs (miRNAs) are small, non-coding RNA molecules that play critical roles in regulating gene expression. They can be found in cells where they modulate the stability and translational efficiency of target mRNAs. Importantly, miRNAs are not only found within cells but can also be detected outside cells in various biological fluids and therefore may not require the harvesting of exosomes. Here's how miRNAs can exist both free-floating and within exosomes:

Encapsulation and Protection: MiRNAs can be packaged into exosomes, which are small vesicles (approximately 30-150 nm in diameter) released by cells into the extracellular environment. The encapsulation in exosomes protects miRNAs from degradation by RNases present in biological fluids, enhancing their stability.

Role in Cell Communication: Exosomal miRNAs are involved in intercellular communication. By transferring miRNAs between cells, exosomes can influence gene expression in recipient cells, thereby modulating cellular behavior and physiological responses.

Biomarker Potential:

Because of their stability and their role in cellular communication, exosomal miRNAs are considered promising biomarkers for various diseases, including cancer, cardiovascular diseases, and neurological disorders. EG. MicroRNA-30 (miR-30) has been identified as a significant biomarker in heart disease. Studies have shown that miR-30 family members, including miR-30a, miR-30b, miR-30c, miR-30d, and miR-30e, are involved in various cardiovascular processes, including cardiac hypertrophy, fibrosis, and myocardial infarction. miR-30 targets and suppresses profibrotic genes, thus preventing the excessive deposition of extracellular matrix proteins and fibrosis in cardiac tissue. Reduced levels of miR-30 are linked to increased fibrosis. [PMID23236408]

Free-Floating MicroRNAs

Direct Release: MiRNAs can also be found free-floating in bodily fluids. These miRNAs may be released from cells through mechanisms other than exosomal packaging, such as apoptosis (cell death) or active secretion.

Binding to Proteins: Some free-floating miRNAs in bodily fluids are associated with protein complexes. For example, miRNAs can bind to Argonaute2 (AGO2), a key protein in the RNA-induced silencing complex (RISC), which protects them from degradation.

Functional Implications: The functional role of free-floating miR-NAs is not as well understood as that of exosomal miRNAs. However, they may still play a role in cell-to-cell communication and could act as biomarkers for disease.

Therefore, MicroRNAs can exist both as free-floating molecules and within exosomes. Each form has its mechanisms of stability and roles in cellular processes and communication. Exosomal miR-NAs, due to their stability and encapsulation, are particularly interesting in the context of disease diagnosis and monitoring, as well as therapeutic applications, such as drug delivery systems. Meanwhile, understanding the roles and mechanisms of free-floating miRNAs continues to be an important area of research in molecular biology and medicine.

The Relationship of miRNA and Cytokine Proteins

MicroRNAs (miRNAs) and cytokines are both critical components in the regulation of cellular processes, especially in the context of immune responses and inflammation. As mentioned, miRNAs are small, non-coding RNA molecules that regulate gene expression at the post-transcriptional level, whereas cytokines are proteins that act as signaling molecules between cells, primarily within the immune system. The relationship between miRNAs and cytokines is complex and involves regulatory interactions where miRNAs can modulate cytokine expression and activity, and vice versa.

Regulation of Cytokine Expression by miRNAs

Targeting mRNA: MiRNAs can directly target the mRNAs of cytokine genes, leading to the degradation of these mRNAs or the inhibition of their translation into proteins. For example, miR-155 is a well-known miRNA that regulates the expression of several inflammatory cytokines.

Influence on Transcription Factors: miRNAs can also influence the expression of cytokines indirectly by targeting transcription factors and other signaling molecules that control cytokine gene transcription. For instance, miR-146a targets signaling proteins such as IRAK1 and TRAF6, which play roles in the NF-κB pathway, a key regulatory pathway of inflammation and cytokine production.

Regulation of miRNA Expression by Cytokines

Cytokine Signaling Inducing miRNA Expression: Cytokine signaling can induce the expression of specific miRNAs. For example, TNF-α and IL-1β can upregulate the expression of miR-146a in various cell types. This miRNA, in turn, can act as a negative feedback regulator to control the signaling pathways that activate these cytokines, thereby modulating the immune response.

Feedback Mechanisms: The interplay between miRNAs and cytokines often involves feedback loops where cytokines regulate the expression of miRNAs that can either promote or inhibit the action of the same or other cytokines. This regulatory mechanism is crucial for maintaining immune homeostasis and preventing excessive inflammatory responses.

Implications in Disease

Inflammatory and Autoimmune Diseases: Dysregulation in the interactions between miRNAs and cytokines can contribute to the pathogenesis of inflammatory and autoimmune diseases. Abnormal miRNA expression can lead to either insufficient or excessive cytokine activity, contributing to disease progression. For example, altered levels of specific miRNAs have been observed in rheumatoid arthritis, multiple sclerosis, and other autoimmune diseases. Jiang 2022: A Four-miRNA-Based Diagnostic Signature for Rheumatoid Arthritis [PMID35251375]

Cancer: In cancer, miRNAs can influence the tumor microenvironment by modulating cytokine production, which can affect tumor growth, metastasis, and the immune response to the tumor. Wang 2022 Identifies microtubule-binding protein CSPP1 as a novel cancer biomarker associated with ferroptosis and tumor microenvironment! [PMID35832625]

In conclusion, the relationship between miRNAs and cytokines is a dynamic and integral part of cellular regulation, particularly in the immune system. Understanding this relationship provides insights into the mechanisms of immune regulation, inflammation, and the pathogenesis of various diseases. It also offers potential therapeutic targets for modulating immune responses and treating inflammatory diseases, cancers, and other conditions where cytokine signaling plays a critical role.

In summary all 'cell-free' preparations of birth tissue pose powerful therapeutic massages in regenerative medicine. Which one of these or in which form or combination will have to be decided in many clinical studies. It is becoming more and more evident that 'cell-free' MSC preparations may be a better clinical choice due to their ease of use, stability and sterility.

miRNA and Immunity

RNA editing, particularly the editing of microRNAs (miRNAs), plays a crucial role in the regulation of gene expression and has significant implications for innate immunity. Here's a detailed look at RNA editing of miRNAs and how it intersects with the body's innate immune response.

RNA Editing of miRNAs- Definition and Mechanisms:

RNA Editing: RNA editing refers to the post-transcriptional modifications of RNA molecules, altering nucleotide sequences and thus affecting their function without changing the underlying DNA. The most common type of RNA editing in mammals is adenosine-to-inosine (A-to-I) editing, mediated by the enzyme family known as ADARs (adenosine deaminases acting on RNA).

miRNA Editing: miRNAs are small non-coding RNAs that regulate gene expression by binding to target messenger RNAs (mRNAs) and typically repressing their translation or promoting their degradation. Editing of miRNAs can alter their maturation, stability, and target specificity.

Impact on miRNA Function - Altered Targeting:

RNA editing can change the sequence of the miRNA seed region, which is critical for target recognition, leading to a different set of target mRNAs being regulated.

Stability and Processing: Editing can affect the processing of primary miRNAs (pri-miRNAs) to precursor miRNAs (pre-miR-

NAs) and mature miRNAs, influencing their stability and abundance.

RNA Editing and Innate Immunity - System Overview:

Innate Immunity: The innate immune system is the body's first line of defense against pathogens, involving physical barriers, immune cells, and various proteins that recognize and respond to foreign invaders.

Role of miRNAs in Immunity: miRNAs are crucial regulators of innate immune responses, modulating the expression of cytokines, receptors, and other signaling molecules involved in immune activation and inflammation.

Influence of RNA Editing on Immunity:

Regulation of Immune Genes: RNA editing of miRNAs can influence the expression of genes involved in the innate immune response. For example, edited miRNAs may have altered affinities for mRNAs encoding cytokines, chemokines, and other immune regulators.

Inflammatory Responses: Editing of miRNAs can impact the production and release of pro-inflammatory and anti-inflammatory cytokines, thereby modulating the inflammatory response. Dysregulation of RNA editing can lead to inappropriate immune activation or suppression.

Examples of RNA Editing in Immunity:

- ADAR1 and Immune Regulation: ADAR1, an enzyme responsible for A-to-I editing, plays a critical role in the innate immune response. It edits both miRNAs and mRNAs, influencing immune signaling pathways. Loss of ADAR1 function can lead to aberrant immune activation and has been implicated in autoimmune diseases and antiviral responses. [PMID34105255, PMID28106799]

- miR-376 Cluster: The miR-376 cluster is a well-studied example where RNA editing significantly alters miRNA function. A-to-I editing in the seed region of miR-376a-1 changes its target specificity, affecting genes involved in immune responses and inflammation. [PMID37967653]

- miR-142: Another example is miR-142, where RNA editing affects its processing and stability. Edited miR-142 has different targets compared to its unedited form, impacting the regulation of immune cell differentiation and function. [PMID37459958]

Clinical and Therapeutic Implications

Autoimmune Diseases: Dysregulation of RNA editing mechanisms can contribute to autoimmune diseases. For instance, insufficient editing by ADAR1 can lead to the accumulation of unedited double-stranded RNAs, triggering inappropriate immune responses and contributing to conditions like Aicardi-Goutières syndrome, a rare genetic disorder that mimics viral infection.

Antiviral Responses: RNA editing plays a critical role in modulating antiviral responses. Edited miRNAs can affect the expression of genes involved in the detection and response to viral infections, potentially influencing the outcome of viral diseases.

Therapeutic Potential: Understanding the role of RNA editing in miRNA function and innate immunity opens up new therapeutic avenues. Modulating RNA editing enzymes like ADAR1 could be a strategy to correct dysregulated immune responses in autoimmune diseases or enhance antiviral defenses.

In summary, RNA editing of miRNAs is a vital post-transcriptional modification process that significantly impacts gene expression and innate immune responses. By altering the sequence and function of miRNAs, RNA editing can influence the regulation of immune genes, inflammatory responses, and the overall immune system's ability to respond to pathogens. Dysregulation of this process can lead to autoimmune diseases and other immune-related conditions, highlighting the importance of RNA editing in maintaining immune homeostasis. Ongoing research in this area holds promise for developing novel therapeutic strategies targeting RNA editing mechanisms to treat immune disorders and enhance antiviral responses.

Key Features Differentiating Self from Non-Self RNA

The innate immune system distinguishes between self and foreign RNA through a combination of pattern recognition receptors (PRRs) and other molecular mechanisms that identify specific features commonly associated with foreign or pathogenic RNA. Here are the primary mechanisms involved [PMID34344870]:

- Pattern Recognition Receptors (PRRs) and Toll-Like Receptors (TLRs):

- TLR3: Recognizes double-stranded RNA (dsRNA), a common viral replication intermediate.

- TLR7/8: Detect single-stranded RNA (ssRNA) typically found in RNA viruses.

- RIG-I-like Receptors (RLRs): Recognizes short double-stranded RNA with a 5' triphosphate end, which is not usually present in mammalian RNA.

- MDA5: Detects long double-stranded RNA, another viral replication product.

- NOD-like Receptors (NLRs): These cytoplasmic receptors detect intracellular pathogens and stress signals, contributing to the detection of foreign RNA.

How does this work?:

5' Triphosphate Group: Most viral RNAs possess a 5' triphosphate group, whereas cellular RNAs are typically capped at the 5' end with a methylated guanine (m^7G cap), distinguishing them from foreign RNAs recognized by RIG-I.

Double-Stranded RNA: While cellular RNA is predominantly single-stranded, many viruses produce double-stranded RNA during replication. TLR3 and MDA5 detect these double-stranded structures.

Uncapped RNA: The presence of uncapped RNA or RNA with unusual cap structures can be a sign of viral origin, detected by receptors like RIG-I.

RNA Modifications: Mammalian RNAs often contain specific modifications (e.g., N^6-methyladenosine, m^6A) that are recognized as self, whereas viral RNAs may lack these modifications or have different patterns.

Mechanisms to Prevent Immune Activation by Self RNA

RNA Editing by ADARs: Adenosine Deaminases Acting on RNA (ADARs) convert adenosine to inosine in dsRNA. This editing can prevent self-RNA from being recognized as foreign by immune sensors like MDA5.

RNA Processing and Compartmentalization: Proper RNA processing, including splicing and modification, and compartmentalization within cellular structures help in distinguishing self from non-self. For example, RNAs in the nucleus are less likely to trigger immune responses compared to cytoplasmic RNAs.

Regulation of PRR Expression and Activation: Cells regulate the expression and activation of PRRs to avoid inappropriate immune responses. For example, PRRs may be more active in cells frequently exposed to pathogens, like immune cells, compared to other cell types.

Examples of Recognition and Response

Viral Infection: Upon viral infection, the presence of viral RNA (with features like 5' triphosphate, lack of capping, and dsRNA) is detected by PRRs like RIG-I, MDA5, and TLRs. This recognition triggers downstream signaling pathways leading to the production of type I interferons and other inflammatory cytokines to combat the infection.

Autoimmune Conditions:

Dysregulation in the mechanisms distinguishing self from non-self RNA can lead to autoimmune diseases. For example, mutations in the ADAR1 gene can cause Aicardi-Goutières syndrome, where unedited self-RNA triggers chronic immune activation.

Thus, The innate immune system uses a sophisticated set of receptors and mechanisms to distinguish between self and foreign RNA. By recognizing specific features commonly associated with pathogenic RNA, such as the 5' triphosphate end and double-stranded structures, and by ensuring that self-RNA is properly modified and processed, the immune system effectively identifies and responds to potential threats while avoiding inappropriate activation against self-RNA. These processes are crucial for maintaining immune homeostasis and preventing autoimmune diseases.

Mesenchymal stem cell (MSC) exosomes, particularly their miRNA content, have shown promise in regenerative medicine due to their ability to modulate immune responses and promote tissue repair. When MSC exosomes are transplanted, their miRNAs can evade the immune response through several mechanisms, ensuring that they deliver their therapeutic effects without being targeted and destroyed by the host's immune system. Here's how MSC exosome miRNAs achieve this:

Immune Evasion by MSC Exosome miRNAs - Surface Protein Composition

Immune-Modulatory Molecules: MSC exosomes often carry surface proteins that help modulate the immune system. For instance, exosomes can express PD-L1 (programmed death-ligand 1), which interacts with PD-1 receptors on immune cells to suppress immune responses.

Self-Markers: Exosomes may carry markers that are recognized as 'self' by the immune system, reducing the likelihood of an immune attack.

Lipid Bilayer Protection: The lipid bilayer of exosomes protects their miRNA cargo from degradation by extracellular RNases and shields them from immune recognition. This ensures that the miRNAs are delivered intact to the target cells.

Targeted Delivery: Exosomes can specifically home to target tissues, reducing exposure to the immune system. This targeted delivery is often mediated by surface proteins and receptors that recognize and bind to specific cell types.

Immune Modulation by Exosomal miRNAs:

Anti-Inflammatory miRNAs: MSC exosomes often contain miRNAs with anti-inflammatory properties. These miRNAs can downregulate pro-inflammatory cytokines and upregulate anti-inflammatory cytokines, creating a local immune-tolerant environment.

Regulation of Immune Cells: Exosomal miRNAs can modulate the activity of immune cells such as macrophages, dendritic cells, and T cells. For example, miRNAs like miR-146a and miR-21 found in MSC exosomes are known to regulate immune responses by targeting key signaling pathways in these cells.

Epigenetic Modulation: MSC exosomal miRNAs can induce epigenetic changes in recipient cells that favor immune tolerance. By altering gene expression profiles, they can promote a regulatory phenotype in immune cells, reducing their reactivity to foreign antigens.

Low Immunogenicity - Lack of MHC Molecules: MSC exosomes typically lack major histocompatibility complex (MHC) molecules, which are critical for antigen presentation and triggering immune responses. This makes them less likely to be recognized as foreign by the host immune system.

Minimal Alloantigen Presentation: Due to the lack of MHC molecules, MSC exosomes present minimal alloantigens, further reducing the risk of eliciting an immune response.

Supporting Studies and Evidence

Study on miR-21 and miR-146a: Research has shown that miR-21 and miR-146a in MSC exosomes play significant roles in modulating immune responses by targeting signaling pathways involved in inflammation and immune activation .

Exosome Surface Proteins: Studies have identified various surface proteins on MSC exosomes that contribute to their immune-modulatory effects, such as PD-L1 and other ligands that interact with immune checkpoints .

Clinical Implications

The ability of MSC exosome miRNAs to evade the immune response has significant implications for their use in therapy. This property enhances the safety and efficacy of MSC exosome-based treatments for a range of conditions, including inflammatory diseases, autoimmune disorders, and tissue regeneration.

Therapeutic Delivery: Ensuring that therapeutic miRNAs are delivered effectively to target tissues without eliciting an immune response improves the potential for MSC exosome-based therapies to achieve their desired outcomes.

Reduced Risk of Rejection: The low immunogenicity of MSC exosomes makes them suitable for allogeneic transplantation, where cells or exosomes from a donor are used to treat a recipient.

In conclusion, MSC exosome miRNAs evade the immune response through a combination of protective mechanisms, including their surface protein composition, lipid bilayer protection, immune-modulatory properties, and low immunogenicity. These features enable MSC exosomes to deliver their therapeutic cargo effectively, promoting tissue repair and modulating immune responses without being targeted by the host's immune system. Understanding these mechanisms is crucial for advancing the clinical application of MSC exosome-based therapies.

motting tissue repair and modulating immune responses within

happ_____ by the host's immune system. Understanding these

mechanisms is crucial for advancing the clinical application of

MSC exosome-based therapies.

Part IV

Applications &
Case Studies

The Emerging Frontiers of MSC Therapy in Medicine

Mesenchymal stem cell (MSC) therapy is heralding a new era in medical treatments, offering unprecedented opportunities for healing and regeneration. The potential applications of MSC therapy are vast and diverse, touching virtually every area of medicine. In this section, we will explore some of the key applications of MSC therapy, with a focus on its current use and emerging potential in various medical fields.

The Broad Spectrum of MSC Applications:

MSC therapy is not limited to a single medical specialty; its applications span a wide range of conditions, from orthopedic injuries to cardiovascular diseases. The versatility of MSCs arises from their ability to differentiate into various cell types, modulate the immune system, and secrete regenerative factors.

Revolutionizing Internal Medicine: Particularly exciting is the use of MSC therapy in internal medicine. The potential to treat acute conditions such as heart attacks and strokes with MSCs is just beginning to be tapped. These therapies could revolutionize the way we approach the treatment of these often-debilitating conditions.

Regulatory Hurdles: Despite the potential benefits, the integration of MSC therapies into mainstream medicine has been slow. One of the significant barriers is regulatory, particularly with institutions like the FDA. The process of approving new medical treatments is rigorous and often lengthy, which can delay the availability of these therapies.

Current 'Shotgun' Approach: Presently, many MSC therapies are applied in a broad, non-specific manner. However, the field is moving towards more targeted and personalized treatments. This includes adjunct therapies that are specific to individual patient needs and post-care that is crucial for maximizing treatment benefits.

The Future of Targeted Therapy:

The next frontier in MSC therapy is the development of targeted treatments for specific organs or tissues. For example, efforts are underway to use MSCs to regenerate insulin-producing beta islet cells in the pancreas for diabetes treatment.

Focus on Osteoarthritis and Orthopedic Repairs: A primary and well-established application of MSC therapy is in the treatment of osteoarthritis and other musculoskeletal conditions, including ligament and tendon repairs. These treatments offer a minimally invasive option compared to traditional surgery and have shown promising results in reducing pain and improving function.

Case Studies and Clinical Evidence: Throughout this section, we will examine a series of case studies and clinical trial results that highlight the effectiveness of MSC therapy in these areas. These real-world examples will provide insight into the practical application and outcomes of MSC treatments in current medical practice.

As we explore these applications, it's important to keep an eye on the future. The field of MSC therapy is rapidly evolving, with ongoing research continually uncovering new potential applications and refining existing treatments.

In conclusion, MSC therapy represents a significant breakthrough in medicine, offering hope for many conditions that were previously difficult to treat. As the field continues to advance, we anticipate a future where MSC therapies are more targeted, efficient, and widely available, fundamentally changing the landscape of medical treatment.

Clinical Applications

We already mentioned a few clinical applications in the chapters above particularly in the area of inflammatory diseases. Here are a few more. Mesenchymal stem cells (MSCs) have a broad range of clinical applications beyond those already discussed, particularly in the treatment of inflammatory diseases. Here's an overview of additional clinical applications that highlight the versatility and potential of MSC therapy in various medical fields:

Neurological Disorders

Stroke: MSC therapy is being investigated for its potential to promote recovery after stroke through neurogenesis, angiogenesis, and modulation of the inflammatory response in the brain.

Multiple Sclerosis (MS): MSCs can modulate the immune system's activity, potentially reducing the autoimmune attack on myelin sheaths in patients with MS, thereby slowing disease progression and alleviating symptoms.

Cardiovascular Diseases

Heart Failure: MSCs can differentiate into cardiac cell types and secrete paracrine factors that promote the repair of damaged heart tissue, potentially improving cardiac function.

Myocardial Infarction: After a heart attack, MSC therapy can help reduce infarct size and restore heart function through regeneration of cardiac tissue and reduction of fibrosis.

Metabolic Disorders

Diabetes: MSCs have the potential to modulate immune responses and protect pancreatic beta cells from autoimmune destruction in type 1 diabetes, and they may help improve insulin sensitivity and pancreatic function in type 2 diabetes. [PMID33995278]

Liver Diseases: MSCs can differentiate into hepatocyte-like cells and provide supportive factors that help repair liver damage in conditions like cirrhosis or chronic hepatitis.

Autoimmune Diseases

Lupus (SLE): By modulating the immune system, MSCs can potentially reduce the severity of systemic lupus erythematosus, a disorder characterized by the immune system attacking its own tissues.

Crohn's Disease: MSCs have been used in clinical trials to treat perianal fistulas in Crohn's disease with promising results, likely due to their ability to modulate inflammation and promote tissue healing.

Orthopedic Conditions

Bone Fractures: MSCs can differentiate into osteoblasts and contribute to the healing of bone fractures and defects by promoting bone regeneration.

Osteoarthritis: As discussed, MSC injections into joint spaces can help alleviate symptoms of osteoarthritis by reducing inflammation and promoting the repair of cartilage.

Dermatological Applications

Wound Healing: MSCs can accelerate wound healing by promoting angiogenesis, modulating inflammation, and enhancing collagen deposition, which is crucial in both acute and chronic wounds.

Scleroderma: For skin conditions like scleroderma, MSCs can modulate the immune response and promote skin regeneration, potentially reducing fibrosis.

In conclusion, the clinical applications of MSCs are vast and varied, reflecting their unique properties of immunomodulation, differentiation potential, and ability to secrete regenerative factors. Ongoing research and clinical trials continue to expand our understanding of how MSCs can be used effectively across a range of conditions, highlighting their potential as a cornerstone of regenerative medicine. As this field evolves, further discoveries will likely unlock new therapeutic possibilities for MSCs in treating complex diseases.

Osteoarthritis and Cartilage Repair in Knees

Currently the most prominent application for MSCs in regenerative Medicine is for Osteoarthritis. In this field many clinical studies and valuable research is available. [PMID34784876, PMID36613502]

An Overview of Osteoarthritis

Osteoarthritis (OA) is a degenerative joint disease, one of the most common forms of arthritis, typically affecting the elderly but can also occur in younger individuals. It is characterized by the breakdown of cartilage—the cushioning material at the end of bones—as well as changes in the bone and deterioration of tendons and ligaments. The primary symptoms include joint pain, stiffness, swelling, and reduced mobility.

Pathophysiology:

- Cartilage Degradation: In OA, the cartilage in the joint breaks down, leading to pain and difficulty in movement.

- Bone Changes: Over time, there may be bone growths (osteophytes) and the underlying bone may also undergo remodeling.

Risk Factors:

- Age: Incidence increases with age.

- Epigenetics: A family history of OA can increase risk.

- Obesity: Extra weight puts more stress on joints, particularly weight-bearing joints like the hips and knees.

- Injury and Overuse: Repeated stress on a joint can lead to OA.

Outcome measures used in patient with knee osteoarthritis

For the purpose of evidence based Medicine it is important to establish measurable outcomes of a treatment is a crucial aspect of clinical research [PMID30842718]. Here are a few reasons why this is important:

- Objective Evaluation: Measurable outcomes provide objective criteria to evaluate the effectiveness of a treatment. Without these metrics, it would be challenging to determine whether a treatment is beneficial.

- Standardization: Having standardized outcome measures allows different studies to be compared and contrasted. This is essential for synthesizing data from multiple sources and for conducting meta-analyses.

- Guiding Clinical Decision-Making: Measurable outcomes help clinicians make informed decisions about the best course of treatment for their patients. They provide evidence-based benchmarks for assessing patient progress.

- Regulatory Approval: Regulatory agencies, such as the FDA or EMA, require evidence of efficacy based on predefined and measurable outcomes to approve new treatments for clinical use.

- Personalized Medicine: In the era of personalized medicine, measurable outcomes can help tailor treatments to individual patients based on their specific response to a therapy.

- Health Economics: Measurable outcomes are also important for assessing the cost-effectiveness of treatments, which is increasingly important in healthcare decision-making.

Types of Measurable Outcomes for OA

- Clinical Endpoints: These include survival rates, disease recurrence, or improvement in symptoms. Clinical endpoints are directly related to patient health and well-being.

- Biomarkers: Biological markers can provide measurable indicators of the biological response to a treatment. For example, a decrease in tumor markers might indicate the effectiveness of a cancer therapy.

- Quality of Life: Assessments of quality of life, including physical, emotional, and social well-being, are increasingly recognized as important outcomes in clinical research.

- Functional Measures: In some cases, functional outcomes such as improved mobility or cognitive function are the primary measures of treatment success.

In summary, establishing and utilizing measurable outcomes in clinical research is fundamental to advancing medical science and improving patient care. It ensures that studies are meaningful, reliable, and contribute to the collective understanding of treatment efficacy.

Here are the measures used in the evaluation of osteoarthritis:

Lequesne Index:

The Lequesne Index is a questionnaire designed to assess the severity of OA. It considers factors like pain or discomfort, maximum distance walked, and activities of daily living. The index is used to evaluate the effectiveness of treatments and the progression of the disease.

WOMAC (Western Ontario and McMaster Universities Osteoarthritis Index):

Purpose: WOMAC is widely used in the clinical evaluation of OA, particularly of the knee and hip. The VAS alone is not sufficient in measuring study outcomes.

WOMAC Components:

- Pain: Assesses pain severity during various activities.

- Stiffness: Measures the degree of joint stiffness.

- Physical Function: Evaluates the difficulty experienced in daily activities.

- Scoring: Patients rate their experiences in these categories, which are then combined for an overall score.

- Visual Analogue Scale (VAS):

- Usage: The VAS is a simple and commonly used method for assessing the intensity of pain.

- Format: It typically consists of a straight line, often 10 centimeters long, where one end signifies 'no pain' and the other 'worst pain imaginable'.

- Scoring: Patients mark a point on the line that corresponds to their perceived pain level.

Traditional vs Treatment Approaches:

Lifestyle Changes: Weight loss, physical therapy, and exercise can help reduce symptoms.

Medications: Pain relievers and anti-inflammatory drugs are commonly used.

Surgical Options: In most cases, joint replacement surgery is the final result of untreated joint degeneration.

Regenerative Approaches to Osteoarthritis

Recent advancements in the treatment of osteoarthritis (OA) have focused on addressing pain, improving joint function, and slowing the progression of the disease. Two notable approaches include injections of peptides and hyaluronic acid:

Peptide Injections

Peptides are increasingly used as stand alone and co-treatment. For the purpose of completeness they should be briefly mentioned here. Specifically standing out is BPC-157, also known as Body Protection Compound-157, is a synthetic peptide that has gained interest for its potential healing and regenerative properties. While it is not yet approved for clinical use, some preclinical studies and anecdotal evidence suggest that it may have beneficial effects for various conditions, including arthritis. Here's what is known so far:

BPC-157 and Arthritis

Anti-inflammatory Effects: BPC-157 has been shown in some animal studies to have anti-inflammatory properties, which could be beneficial in reducing the inflammation associated with arthritis.

Tissue Healing: The peptide is believed to promote the healing of various tissues, including tendons, ligaments, and muscle. This could potentially aid in the repair of damaged joint tissues in arthritis.

Angiogenesis: BPC-157 may promote angiogenesis, the formation of new blood vessels, which can improve blood flow and nutrient delivery to arthritic joints, potentially aiding in the healing process.

Cartilage Protection: Some studies suggest that BPC-157 could have a protective effect on cartilage, which is often degraded in arthritic conditions.

Considerations and Limitations

Limited Research: Most of the research on BPC-157 has been conducted in animal models, and there is limited clinical data on its efficacy and safety in humans, particularly for the treatment of arthritis.

Regulatory Status: BPC-157 is not currently approved by regulatory agencies like the FDA for the treatment of arthritis or any other condition.

Safety Concerns: The long-term safety and potential side effects of BPC-157, especially when used for chronic conditions like arthritis, are not well understood.

Availability: Due to its unapproved and controlled FDA status, BPC-157 is primarily available as a research chemical, and its quality and purity may vary.

General Mechanism of Peptide Action:

Peptides are short chains of amino acids that can mimic the action of natural growth factors or signaling molecules in the body. In the context of OA, certain peptides may promote cartilage repair, reduce inflammation, and alleviate pain.

Types of Peptides: Research is ongoing to identify specific peptides that are effective in treating OA. Some studies have focused on peptides that can stimulate the regeneration of cartilage or modulate the inflammatory response.

Clinical Trials: While peptide-based therapies for OA are still in the early stages of development, some clinical trials have shown promising results in terms of pain reduction and improved joint function.

Hyaluronic Acid Injections

Hyaluronic acid (HA) is a naturally occurring glycosaminoglycan, which is a type of long-chain carbohydrate molecule. It is found in various tissues throughout the body, including the skin, eyes, and joint fluid. Hyaluronic acid plays a crucial role in maintaining the hydration, elasticity, and structural integrity of these tissues. Here are some key points about hyaluronic acid:

Properties and Functions of Hyaluronic Acid

Hydration: Hyaluronic acid can retain a significant amount of water (up to 1,000 times its weight), making it an essential component for maintaining tissue hydration and lubrication.

Viscoelasticity: In joint fluid, hyaluronic acid contributes to the viscoelastic properties that provide lubrication and shock absorption, protecting joints during movement.

Wound Healing: HA is involved in various stages of wound healing, including inflammation, granulation, and tissue remodeling. It helps regulate the migration and proliferation of cells necessary for tissue repair.

Skin Health: In the skin, hyaluronic acid helps maintain moisture, firmness, and elasticity. It is a critical component of the extracellular matrix that supports skin structure.

Clinical and Cosmetic Applications

Osteoarthritis Treatment: Hyaluronic acid injections, known as viscosupplementation, are used to treat knee osteoarthritis by improving joint lubrication and reducing pain.

Dermal Fillers: In cosmetic dermatology, HA-based dermal fillers are used to reduce the appearance of wrinkles, add volume to facial features, and enhance skin hydration.

Eye Surgery: Hyaluronic acid is used as a viscoelastic agent in eye surgeries, including cataract surgery, to maintain the shape of the eye and protect delicate tissues.

Skin Care Products: Many skin care products, including serums and moisturizers, contain hyaluronic acid for its hydrating and anti-aging properties.

Hyaluronic acid is a versatile and essential molecule with a wide range of functions in the body, particularly in maintaining hydration and elasticity in tissues. Its unique properties have made it valuable in medical and cosmetic applications, from treating joint disorders to enhancing skin health and appearance.

Viscosupplementation:

Hyaluronic acid injections, also known as viscosupplementation, involve injecting hyaluronic acid directly into the joint space. Hyaluronic acid is a natural component of joint fluid and cartilage, and it helps to lubricate and cushion the joint.

Pain Relief and Improved Mobility: These injections can provide pain relief and improve joint mobility for patients with OA. The effects can last for several months, although the efficacy may vary among individuals.

Clinical Use: Hyaluronic acid injections are commonly used for knee osteoarthritis, and they are generally considered safe with minimal side effects. However, their effectiveness compared to other treatments, such as corticosteroid injections, is still a subject of debate in the medical community and Hyaluronic acid injections are often used as a negative control in studies.

Recent advancements in the treatment of osteoarthritis, including peptide and hyaluronic acid injections, offer new avenues for managing this chronic condition. While hyaluronic acid injections are already widely used in clinical practice, peptide-based therapies are an emerging area of research with potential for future applications. As our understanding of OA and its underlying mechanisms continues to evolve, these and other innovative treatments hold promise for improving the quality of life for individuals affected by osteoarthritis.

In summary, Osteoarthritis is a chronic condition that significantly impacts quality of life. Accurately measuring its severity and treatment outcomes is crucial for effective management. Tools like the Lequesne Index, WOMAC, and VAS provide standardized methods for assessing these factors, aiding in both clinical research and patient care.

Emerging 'stem cell' therapy alternatives for OA

How do you know that your therapy is effective? You establish measurable markers and standards and subject them to scrutiny in randomized controlled clincal studies. The evaluation of therapy efficacy in osteoarthritis (OA) is crucial to determine whether a treatment with MSCs is truly working. Without reliable and standardized evaluation methods, it would be challenging to objectively assess improvement or progression of the disease. These methods take into account both subjective patient-reported outcomes and objective clinical data.

Measurable Data in Therapy Assessment:- T2-MRI Quantification:

Purpose: Magnetic Resonance Imaging (MRI) with T2 mapping is used to assess the health of cartilage. T2 relaxation times are sensitive to changes in the water content and collagen structure of cartilage, which are indicative of OA.

Relevance: By quantifying changes in the T2 relaxation time, clinicians can objectively evaluate the structural changes in the joint, providing a clear picture of the therapy's impact on joint health.

WOMAC Index:

As mentioned above, the Western Ontario and McMaster Universities Osteoarthritis Index (WOMAC) is a detailed, validated questionnaire specifically designed for assessing the condition of patients with OA of the knee and hip.

Components of the WOMAC score in detail:

- Pain (5 items): Assesses pain severity during various activities like walking, using stairs, in bed, sitting or lying, and standing upright.

- Stiffness (2 items): Evaluates the degree of stiffness after waking up and later in the day.

- Physical Function (17 items): Measures difficulty in daily activities such as walking, getting in/out of a car, shopping, putting on socks, etc.

- Scoring: Each item is scored, allowing clinicians to quantify the severity of symptoms and functional limitations. This provides a comprehensive view of the patient's condition and the impact of the treatment.

Importance of MRI Methods:

Objective Assessment: Tools like T2 MRI provide objective data, crucial for corroborating patient-reported outcomes.

Standardization: Standardized tools like WOMAC ensure that the data collected are reliable and comparable across different studies or treatment regimens.

Treatment Adjustment: These evaluation methods allow clinicians to monitor the effectiveness of a therapy and make necessary adjustments for optimal patient care.

Research and Development: In clinical research, these tools are essential for assessing the efficacy of new treatments, contributing to evidence-based practice.

To summarize, In the treatment of OA, the combination of subjective assessments (like WOMAC) and objective measurements (like T2 MRI quantification) offers a comprehensive approach to evaluating therapy effectiveness. This balanced evaluation is essential not only for clinical decision-making but also for advancing research in the field, ultimately leading to more effective and personalized treatment strategies for OA.

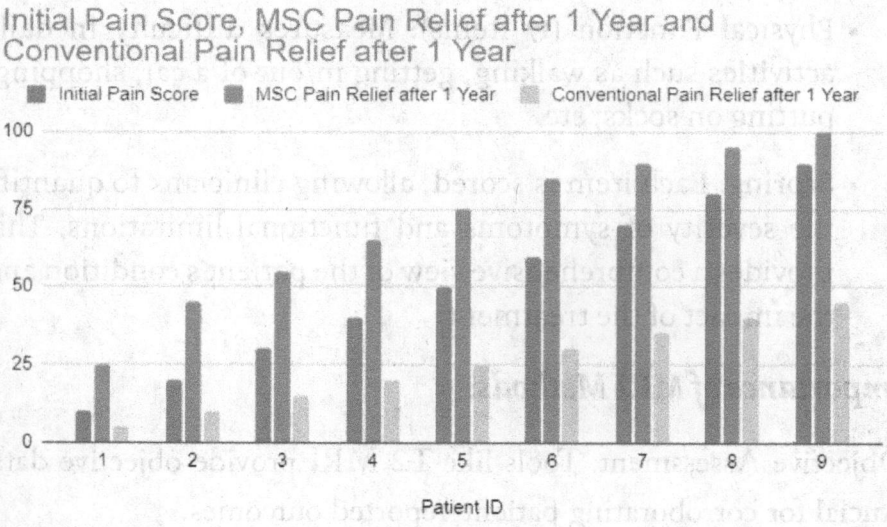

Initial Pain Score, MSC Pain Relief after 1 Year and Conventional Pain Relief after 1 Year

■ Initial Pain Score   ■ MSC Pain Relief after 1 Year   ▨ Conventional Pain Relief after 1 Year

Fig.13: Orozco shows how MSC treatment was superior to conventional treatments (adopted from Lluis Orozco 2013 [PMID23680930].

"The worse the injury, the better the outcome!"

Here are examples of clinical studies which quantify the outcome of MSC therapies in Osteoarthritis. This excellent study particularly stands out as it includes all the measures discussed above.

Fig.14 adopted from Lluis Orozco (2013) shows: 'the worse the initial poor cartilage score was the better the outcome'. Twelve patients were followed over 1 year. WOMAC, Lequesne and VAS scores were recorded. Cartilage quality was assessed by MRI-T2 mapping and was quantified as the PCI (poor cartilage index). [PMID23680930]

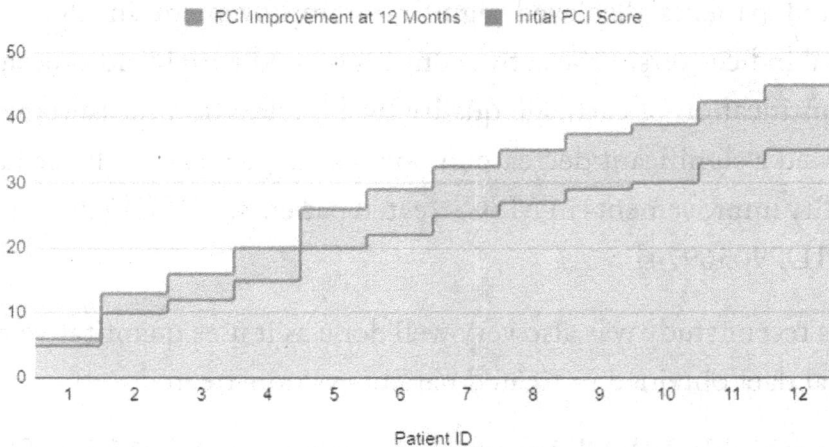

Initial PCI Score and PCI Improvement at 12 Months

Fig.14: "the worse the initial PCI (poor cartilage index) was in patients – the better the outcome" (adopted from Lluis Orozco 2013, PMID23680930).

These Results were also reaffirmed after a 2 year follow up. [PMID24887752]. The health assessment questionnaire revealed a significant improvement in all patients. Moreover, T2-MRI mapping showed signs of cartilage regeneration in all patients at 12 months post-treatment. [PMID26783191]

Soler 2016: "The MSC-treated patients displayed significant improvement in algofunctional indices versus the active controls treated with hyaluronic acid. Quantification of cartilage quality by T2 relaxation measurements showed a significant decrease in poor cartilage areas, with cartilage quality improvements in MSC-treated patients. No pathological values were found at 12 months in previously healthy areas, therefore no progression of OA degeneration was observed." [PMID26783191]

Vega2015: "We randomized 30 patients with chronic knee pain unresponsive to conservative treatments and showed radiological evidence of osteoarthritis into 2 groups of 15 patients. The MSC-treated patients displayed significant improvement in algofunctional indices versus the active controls treated with hyaluronic acid. Quantification of cartilage quality by T2 relaxation measurements showed a significant decrease in poor cartilage areas, with cartilage quality improvements in MSC-treated patients." [PMID25822648, PMID29056974]

This recent study was also very well done as it uses quantitative and visual data obtained in treated patients vs non-treated:

Quantifiable MRI T2 mapping Turajane et al. 2017 key findings Total WOMAC score was reduced 70% after 12 Month compared to 40% in "control group". TKA was necessary in 3 patients in control group 3 while none in group 1 or 2. =>

group 3 control showed no improvement. There were no notable adverse events. [PMID29056974]

Jeyaraman (2022) reports a meta analyses: "In total, 21 studies with a total of 936 patients were analyzed - Although both allogeneic and autologous sources of MSCs demonstrated significantly better VAS improvement after 6 months , this trend was not maintained after 1 year for the allogeneic source. When compared to their respective controls based on WOMAC scores after 1 year, autologous sources of MSCs performed better than allogeneic sources although the author admits there was a significant amount of heterogeneity among the included studies. As a result, the random-effects model was used in the analysis at all time points and that publication bias is at a minimum level." In other words, comparing apples to oranges due to challenges in evaluating allogeneic MSC sources and their quality is and remains a challenge. [PMID36507199]

Kim (2023) shows actual arthroscopic images of cartilage growth that unfortunately cannot be reproduced here. "Improved clinical and radiological outcomes and favorable cartilage regeneration were seen after surgery for varus Knee OA in both SVF and hUCB-MSC groups. We think that no significant differences were found in ICRS grades between the groups, which indicated that SVF implantation could obtain cartilage regeneration as favorable as hUCB-MSC transplantation." This study made an effort to compare apples and oranges: "In this study, an average of 76 million SVF cells, which contained an average of 7.2 million stem cells, were used for SVF implantation, and 7.5×106 cord blood–derived MSCs were used for hUCB-MSC transplantation. [PMID37388880]

Summary of Effects – MSC vs Traditional TKA

Knee osteoarthritis (OA) is a chronic condition that leads to joint pain, stiffness, and decreased mobility. Traditional treatments have predominantly centered around Total Knee Arthroplasty (TKA), which, although effective in relieving symptoms, involves invasive surgery and entails significant recovery time. Conversely, emerging treatments like Mesenchymal Stem Cells (MSC) therapy have shown promise as a less invasive option that potentially enhances cartilage repair and improves joint function.

Study Outcomes on MSC Treatment:

Recent studies focusing on the efficacy of MSC treatment for knee OA reveal significant improvements in cartilage quality and joint function. Data, such as that from MRI T2 mapping, quantifies this improvement using the Poor Cartilage Index (PCI), which shows how MSC therapy leads to a notable decrease in PCI scores over time, indicating better cartilage health. For instance, consistent reductions in PCI were statistically significant at 6, 9, and 12 months post-intervention, illustrating ongoing improvement.

Additionally, the correlation between initial PCI scores and the extent of improvement after 12 months further supports the efficacy of MSC treatments. Higher initial PCI scores corresponded to more significant improvements, suggesting that even patients with severe cartilage degradation could benefit from MSC therapy.

Comparison with Traditional TKA:

Traditional TKA effectively alleviates pain and restores function but involves replacing the knee joint with artificial components. While TKA is a well-established solution for end-stage knee OA, it comes with the risks of surgery, a lengthy rehabilitation process, and potential complications such as infection and prosthesis wear and loosening.

In contrast to TKA, MSC treatments offer a regenerative approach, aiming to repair the damaged cartilage inherently. The advantages of MSC over TKA include:

1) Minimally invasive procedure: MSC therapy involves injections, which are less invasive than knee replacement surgery.

2) Potential for natural cartilage repair: MSCs have regenerative properties that may facilitate the natural healing of cartilage, rather than replacing it.

3) Shorter recovery time: Patients typically experience a quicker return to daily activities after MSC injections compared to TKA recovery.

4) Lower risk of complications: Being less invasive, MSC therapy carries a lower risk of surgical complications.

In Conclusion, the comparative analysis of MSC therapy versus traditional TKA for treating knee OA highlights MSC's potential advantages in terms of invasiveness, natural healing, and recovery. The significant improvements in cartilage quality and joint functionality underscore MSC therapy as a promising alternative for patients seeking less invasive treatments. While TKA remains a viable option for severe and end-stage knee OA, MSC treatments offer a hopeful future for regenerative joint therapies, potentially shifting the treatment paradigm in orthopedics. Further long-term studies and clinical trials will be critical to fully understand the benefits, limitations, and clinical applications of MSC therapy in knee OA.

ACL and Meniscus Repair

Introduction: The anterior cruciate ligament (ACL) and the meniscus are critical structures in the knee that are prone to injuries, especially in athletes and active individuals. Traditional repair techniques, such as surgical reconstruction for the ACL and meniscectomy or meniscal repair for the meniscus, though effective, have limitations including long recovery periods, risk of complications, and in some cases, the onset of osteoarthritis later in life. Mesenchymal Stem Cells (MSC) therapy represents a burgeoning field that aims to enhance the regenerative capabilities of these tissues, potentially offering improved outcomes with fewer long-term complications.

Mechanisms of MSC in ACL and Meniscus Repair:

MSC therapy works by exploiting the regenerative properties of stem cells, which can differentiate into various types of cells, including osteocytes, chondrocytes, and fibroblasts. This ability is particularly beneficial for:

ACL Repair: MSCs can promote the formation of fibrocartilaginous tissue, improving the structural and functional properties of the ligament.

Meniscus Repair: MSCs contribute to the generation of new cartilage cells and extracellular matrix, which are essential for restoring the meniscus's cushioning and load-bearing functions.

Clinical Evidence and Outcomes:

Emerging clinical trials and studies on MSC therapy for ACL and meniscus injuries have shown promising results:

Improved Healing: MSCs enhance the biological healing processes, potentially leading to stronger, more durable repairs.

Reduced Recovery Time: Early evidence suggests that MSC treatment may accelerate the healing process, enabling quicker rehabilitation and return to activity.

Decreased Re-Injury Rates: By promoting more natural healing and possibly restoring the native anatomy and biomechanics better than traditional methods, MSC therapy could reduce the likelihood of re-injury.

Preservation of Joint Health: MSC therapy may help preserve the joint's biomechanics, reducing the risk of osteoarthritis development compared to traditional surgical approaches.

Current Challenges and Considerations:

While the use of MSC for ACL and meniscus repair is exciting, several challenges need addressing to realize its full potential:

Standardization of Treatment Protocols: There is a need for standardized protocols regarding MSC preparation, delivery, and post-treatment rehabilitation.

Long-term Safety and Efficacy: Longitudinal studies are essential to assess the long-term safety and effectiveness of MSC treatments in ACL and meniscus repair.

Studies on Meniscus repair:

- Whitehouse MR 2017: Repair of Torn Avascular Meniscal Cartilage Using Undifferentiated Autologous Mesenchymal

Stem Cells: From In Vitro Optimization to a First-in-Human Study. Stem Cells Transl Med. 2017 Apr;6(4):1237-1248. [PMID28186682]

- Zhou YF, Zhang D, Yan WT, Lian K, Zhang ZZ. Meniscus Regeneration With Multipotent Stromal Cell Therapies. Front Bioeng Biotechnol. 2022 Feb 9;10:796408. doi: 10.3389/fbioe.2022.796408. [PMID: 35237572]

- Chen Z, Jin M, He H, Dong J, Li J, Nie J, Wang Z, Xu J, Wu F. Mesenchymal stem cells and macrophages and their interactions in tendon-bone healing. "As the 'sensor and switch of the immune system', mesenchymal stem cells (MSCs) respond to the inflammatory environment and exert immunomodulatory effects during the tendon-bone healing process." J Orthop Translat. 2023 Jan 20;39:63-73. doi: 10.1016/j.jot.2022.12.005. PMID: 37188000; PMCID: PMC10175706.

In conclusion, MSC therapy offers a promising adjunct or alternative to traditional surgical methods for ACL and meniscus repair. The potential for enhanced tissue regeneration, reduced recovery time, and lower re-injury rates positions MSC as a transformative approach in orthopedic medicine. However, further research is essential to optimize protocols, confirm long-term benefits, and integrate MSC therapy into standard clinical practice. As the body of evidence grows, MSC could significantly impact how ACL and meniscus injuries are treated, emphasizing restoration and preservation over mere repair.

Co-injection of Peptides BPC-157, TGF-beta1 and Hyaluronic Acid: Therapeutic Implications

BPC-157 and Hyaloronic acid were already mentioned above. Here are a few more details on their mechanism. BPC-157 has garnered attention for its potential healing properties, particularly in soft tissue repair. It is derived from a protein found in stomach juice and is believed to promote tissue healing and regeneration. Hyaluronic acid, a naturally occurring substance in the body, is known for its role in maintaining moisture and lubrication in the skin and joints, and is commonly used in treatments for osteoarthritis and dermal fillers. The co-injection of these two compounds—BPC-157 for its regenerative capabilities and hyaluronic acid for its lubricating properties—presents a novel approach for enhancing joint and soft tissue repair.

Transforming Growth Factor-beta1 (TGF-ß1) is a critical cytokine involved in the regulation of cell growth, proliferation, differentiation, and apoptosis. It plays a significant role in wound healing and the maintenance of tissue homeostasis. TGF-ß1 is part of the MSC secretome as mentioned many times above. It is a larger protein but can be synthesized using recombinant DNA technology, where the gene encoding TGF-ß1 is inserted into a bacterial, yeast, or mammalian cell line, which then produces the protein. The addition of TGF-ß1 to BPC-157 and hyaluronic acid could potentiate the therapeutic effects of these agents in regenerative medicine, particularly in the healing of joint and soft tissue injuries.

Mechanisms of Action:

TGF-ß1:

- Stimulates the production of extracellular matrix components such as collagen, fibronectin, and proteoglycans, essential for tissue repair.
- Modulates the inflammatory response, promoting a healing environment that can reduce chronic inflammation and facilitate quicker recovery,
- Influences cellular migration and angiogenesis, essential for effective tissue regeneration.

BPC-157:

- Promotes cell survival and angiogenesis (formation of new blood vessels).
- Enhances the healing of tendons, ligaments, and even bones.
- Demonstrates protective effects against damage caused by NSAIDs (non-steroidal anti-inflammatory drugs) on the gut lining.
- Positively influences the nitric oxide (NO) system, which plays a pivotal role in healing and regeneration.

Hyaluronic Acid:

- Acts as a lubricant and shock absorber in the joints.
- Facilitates the transport of nutrients to the cells and the removal of waste products.
- Exhibits anti-inflammatory properties by modulating the activity of various inflammatory markers.
- Enhances the viscoelastic properties of joint fluid, improving joint function and reducing pain.

Clinical Applications and Benefits:

The combination of BPC-157 and hyaluronic acid could be particularly beneficial in the following clinical scenarios:

Joint Disorders: Effective in managing symptoms of osteoarthritis, including pain and stiffness. Hyaluronic acid improves joint lubrication, while BPC-157 may enhance the underlying tissue repair.

Soft Tissue Injuries: Useful in the treatment of muscle, ligament, and tendon injuries where BPC-157 can accelerate healing, and hyaluronic acid can reduce joint-related complications post-injury.

Surgical Recovery: Could be applied postoperatively to enhance tissue healing and expedite recovery, especially in joint surgeries like ACL reconstruction or meniscal repair.

Research and Evidence: Although individual studies have supported the benefits of BPC-157 and hyaluronic acid, research on their combined effects remains limited. Preliminary studies and anecdotal evidence suggest that their synergistic effects could enhance therapeutic outcomes, but more rigorous clinical trials are needed to substantiate these claims and to establish optimal dosing regimens.

Challenges and Considerations:

Regulatory Status: BPC-157, like many other peptides is not currently approved by bodies like the FDA for clinical use, poses a challenge for its adoption in standardized medical practice.

Long-term Effects: Longitudinal studies are needed to understand the long-term implications of co-injecting these compounds, especially concerning potential side effects and the sustainability of therapeutic effects.

Cost and Accessibility: The relatively low cost of these treatments and their availability to patients are also crucial factors that will determine the feasibility of widespread clinical use.

In conclusion, the co-injection of BPC-157 and hyaluronic acid represents a promising but relatively unexplored treatment strategy for enhancing joint health and expediting recovery from soft tissue injuries. While the theoretical benefits of this combination are supported by the properties of each compound, further empirical evidence is required to fully integrate such treatments into routine clinical protocols. Healthcare professionals and researchers should focus on designing controlled clinical trials to evaluate the efficacy and safety of this innovative approach.

Spinal Disc Injuries and the Potential of Stem Cell Therapy

Spinal disc injuries are among the most painful and debilitating medical conditions, significantly impacting an individual's quality of life. These injuries can range from disc herniation and degeneration to severe cases of trauma that may lead to paralysis. Traditional surgical interventions, such as laminectomy, often provide only temporary relief and can sometimes exacerbate the problem by placing additional stress on adjacent discs. In contrast, modern stem cell therapy offers a promising solution for long-term healing, even in the most severely damaged disc joints.

Traditional Treatments and Their Limitations

Laminectomy and Other Surgeries: Surgical procedures like laminectomy involve removing part of the vertebra to relieve pressure on the spinal cord or nerves. While this can provide immediate pain relief, it often fails to address the underlying degeneration of the disc and can lead to further issues. Over time, patients may experience recurring pain as adjacent discs bear the additional load, potentially leading to further degeneration and need for additional surgeries.

Conservative Treatments: Non-surgical treatments such as physical therapy, pain management medications, and epidural steroid injections can help manage symptoms but do not address the root cause of disc degeneration. These treatments often provide only temporary relief and do not contribute to the regeneration of the damaged disc tissue.

The Promise of Stem Cell Therapy

Regenerative Potential: Stem cells, particularly mesenchymal stem cells (MSCs), have the ability to differentiate into various cell types, including those found in spinal discs. When injected into the damaged disc, these stem cells can promote the regeneration of disc tissue, potentially restoring the disc's structure and function.

Anti-inflammatory Effects: MSCs also have powerful anti-inflammatory properties. They can modulate the immune response, reducing inflammation and pain associated with disc injuries. This helps create a more favorable environment for healing and regeneration.

Long-term Healing: Unlike surgical interventions that often only provide temporary relief, stem cell therapy aims to heal the disc itself. By regenerating the damaged tissue, stem cell therapy can provide long-lasting improvements in pain and function, reducing the need for repeated treatments or surgeries.

Minimally Invasive: Stem cell therapy is a minimally invasive procedure, typically involving the injection of stem cells into the affected disc under imaging guidance. This approach reduces the risks associated with major surgery and has a shorter recovery time.

Clinical Evidence, Innovations and Success Rate

The main root cause of DDD (degenerative disc disease) is chronic inflammation due to omega-3 deficiency. Even if traumatic injuries are the etiology, the healing process can never smooth at a 30:1 omega6/3 inflammatory index. Before this root deficiency is addressed years go by. Meanwhile, MSC injections are the fastest and non-invasive treatment available. Research and clinical trials have shown promising results for stem cell therapy in treating spinal disc injuries. Fig. 15 shows patients have reported significant improvements in pain, mobility, and overall quality of life. Studies have demonstrated that stem cell therapy can lead to the regeneration of disc tissue, reducing the need for further surgical interventions.

Kumar 2017: "VAS, ODI, and SF-36 scores significantly improved in both groups receiving both low and high cell doses, and did not differ significantly between the two groups. [PMID29141662]

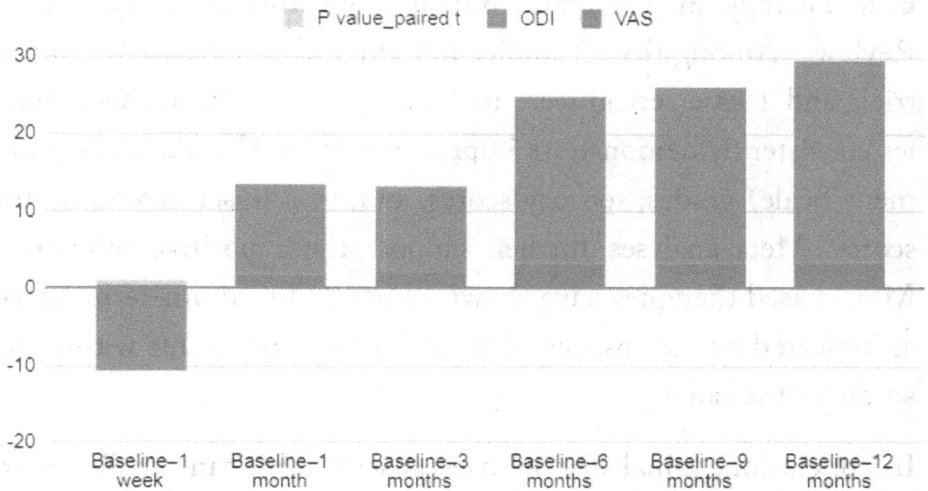

Fig.15: VAS – visual analogue scale, ODI – Oswestry Disability Index (improvements by points); data adopted from [PMID29141662]

Spinal Paralysis

There are many anecdotal reports of successful reversing spinal traumatic paralysis cases. They are available now from testimonials of renowned clinicians. Some clinical studies are also available. Here is an example of a phase I clinical trial:

Bydon M, et al 2024 "Intrathecal delivery of adipose-derived mesenchymal stem cells in traumatic spinal cord injury: Phase I trial. - At final follow-up, seven patients demonstrated improvement in AIS grade from the time of injection. In conclusion, the study met the primary endpoint, demonstrating that AD-MSC harvesting and administration were well-tolerated in patients with traumatic SCI. Nat Commun. 2024 [PMID: 38561341]

Montoto-Meijide 2023 [PMID: 37511478]; "Mesenchymal Stem Cell Therapy in Traumatic Spinal Cord Injury: A Systematic Review - Among the 53 studies initially identified, 22 (21 clinical trials and 1 case series) were included. Findings from these studies consistently demonstrate improvements in AIS (ASIA Impairment Scale) grades, sensory scores, and, to a lesser extent, motor scores. Meta-analyses further support these positive outcomes. MSC-based therapies have shown short- and medium-term safety, as indicated by the absence of significant adverse events within the studied timeframe."

In conclusion, spinal disc injuries pose a significant challenge to long-term health and well-being, often resulting in chronic pain and disability. While traditional treatments like laminectomy provide temporary relief, they do not address the underlying issues of disc degeneration. Stem cell therapy, with its regenerative and anti-inflammatory properties, offers a promising alternative that can lead to long-term healing and improvement in quality of life. As research and clinical applications continue to advance, stem cell therapy holds the potential to revolutionize the treatment of spinal disc injuries, offering hope to those suffering from these debilitating conditions.

Applications for Internal Medicine

Internal Medicine applications for stem cell therapy are beyond the scope of this book. This field is also rapidly advancing in both research and clinic. Stem cell therapy has shown potential in treating various conditions within internal medicine, ranging from autoimmune diseases to degenerative conditions. Below are just a few examples.of clinical applications of stem cell therapies for different diseases.

Stem cell therapy has shown potential in treating various conditions within internal medicine. It's important to distinguish between natural mesenchymal stem cells (MSCs), which offer a broad "shotgun" approach, and targeted stem cell therapies involving induced pluripotent stem cells (iPSCs) and genetically modified stem cells, which provide more specific and directed treatment options.

Natural MSCs as a "Shotgun" Approach"

Broad Application: MSCs can be sourced from bone marrow, adipose tissue, and umbilical cord blood, among other tissues. They are known for their anti-inflammatory and immunomodulatory properties, making them suitable for a wide range of conditions.

Mechanisms: As explained above, MSCs work through paracrine signaling, releasing bioactive molecules that promote tissue repair and modulate immune responses. Their effects are broad and non-specific, which can be beneficial in systemic conditions such as autoimmune diseases.

Examples: MSCs are used in treating rheumatoid arthritis, heart disease, stroke, diabetes, and COPD, where their regenerative and anti-inflammatory properties help improve clinical outcomes.

Targeted iPSCs and Genetically Modified Stem Cells

Precision Therapy: iPSCs are generated by reprogramming adult cells to a pluripotent state, allowing them to differentiate into any cell type. This ability enables the development of patient-specific therapies that precisely target the underlying causes of diseases.

Genetic Modification: Genetically modified stem cells can be engineered to express specific genes, enhancing their therapeutic potential. This approach allows for targeted treatment of genetic disorders and more precise intervention in disease pathways.

Examples: iPSCs are being explored for regenerative applications in cardiac and neural tissues, offering potential cures for conditions like heart disease and neurodegenerative disorders. Genetically modified stem cells are used in gene therapy for diseases such as sickle cell anemia and certain cancers.

While natural MSCs provide a versatile and broadly applicable treatment option, targeted therapies using iPSCs and genetically modified stem cells offer precision and specificity, addressing specific disease mechanisms more effectively. The choice between these approaches in the present and future depends on the condition being treated, the desired therapeutic outcomes, and the individual patient's needs.

Clinical trials are available for both natural MSC therapies and targeted iPS and genetically modified stem cell therapies. To explore current and upcoming clinical trials, you can search databases like ClinicalTrials.gov for the latest information on stem cell therapies. These databases provide detailed information about ongoing studies, eligibility criteria, locations, and study results. Here are examples of clinical trials for each:

Natural MSC Therapies

Rheumatoid Arthritis: Clinical trials have demonstrated that MSC therapy can reduce inflammation and improve joint function in RA patients.

Heart Disease: Trials such as CADUCEUS have shown that MSCs can improve cardiac function and reduce scar tissue post-myocardial infarction.

COPD: Early-phase clinical trials indicate that MSC therapy can reduce inflammation and improve lung function in COPD patients.

Targeted iPS and Genetically Modified Stem Cells

iPSCs for Cardiac Repair: Clinical trials are investigating the use of iPSCs to regenerate cardiac tissue and improve heart function after myocardial infarction.

Gene Therapy for Sickle Cell Disease: Trials using genetically modified stem cells have shown promising results in curing sickle cell disease by correcting the genetic defect in hematopoietic stem cells.

Neurodegenerative Disorders: iPSC-based therapies are being explored for their potential to regenerate neural tissues and improve outcomes in conditions like Parkinson's disease and ALS.

Both natural MSC therapies and targeted iPS and genetically modified stem cell therapies are actively being investigated in clinical trials, highlighting their potential to address a wide range of medical conditions. The choice of therapy depends on the specific disease, the desired outcomes, and patient-specific factors, with ongoing research continually enhancing our understanding and application of these advanced treatments.

Examples of Clinical Applications:

1. Rheumatoid Arthritis (RA)

Probably one of the most prominent internal medicine applications for stem cells are autoimmunity and namely RA.

Therapy: Mesenchymal stem cells (MSCs) Mechanism: MSCs modulate the immune response and reduce inflammation, potentially halting the progression of RA and promoting the repair of damaged tissues. Clinical Evidence: Studies have demonstrated that MSCs can reduce symptoms and improve quality of life in RA patients by reducing inflammatory cytokines and promoting tissue repair.

Mesenchymal Stem Cells (MSCs): MSCs have been shown to reduce inflammation and modulate the immune response in RA patients, providing relief from symptoms and improving quality of life. Clinical trials have reported significant improvements in pain and function, with a stable clinical response observed up to three years post-treatment.

Sarsenova 2021: "Mesenchymal Stem Cell-Based Therapy for Rheumatoid Arthritis" [PMID34769021]

Mesa et al., 2023, "Safety and efficacy of mesenchymal stem cells therapy in the treatment of rheumatoid arthritis" in PLOS One. [PMID37498842]

Lopez-Santalla et al., 2023, "Mesenchymal stem/stromal cell-based therapy for the treatment of rheumatoid arthritis" in The Lancet. [PMID34161884]

Luque-Campos et al., 2019 "Mesenchymal Stem Cells Improve Rheumatoid Arthritis Progression by Controlling Memory T Cell Response - Indeed, given the plasticity of memory CD4+ T cells, it is reasonable to think that MSCs will restore the balance between pro-inflammatory and anti-inflammatory memory T cells populations deregulated in RA leading to prompt their therapeutic function." [PMID31040848]

Mebarki M. et al., 2021 "Development of a human umbilical cord-derived mesenchymal stromal cell-based advanced therapy medicinal product to treat immune and/or inflammatory diseases " [PMID34774107]

2. Heart Disease and Stroke

Therapy: MSCs and cardiac stem cells Mechanism: Stem cells can promote angiogenesis, reduce apoptosis, and regenerate damaged heart tissue following myocardial infarction (heart attack) and ischemic stroke. Clinical Evidence: Trials such as the BOOST and CADUCEUS trials have shown improvements in cardiac function and reduction in infarct size after stem cell therapy.

Cardiac Stem Cells: Studies have demonstrated that MSCs and cardiac stem cells can promote angiogenesis, reduce apoptosis, and regenerate damaged heart tissue. Clinical trials, such as the BOOST and CADUCEUS trials, have shown improvements in cardiac function and reduction in infarct size after stem cell therapy.

3. Diabetes

Therapy: MSCs and pancreatic islet cells Mechanism: MSCs modulate the immune response and promote the regeneration of pancreatic islet cells, improving insulin production and glycemic control. Clinical Evidence: Early clinical trials have shown that stem cell therapy can reduce insulin dependence in type 1 diabetes and improve glycemic control in type 2 diabetes. [PMID33995278]

Pancreatic Islet Cells and MSCs: Stem cell therapy aims to regenerate pancreatic islet cells, improving insulin production and glycemic control. Early clinical trials have shown promising results in reducing insulin dependence in type 1 diabetes and improving glycemic control in type 2 diabetes.

Eleonora de Klerk 2021 "Stem Cell-Based Clinical Trials for Diabetes Mellitus" [PMID33716982]

Barachini 2023 "Mesenchymal Stem Cell in Pancreatic Islet Transplantation" [PMID37239097]

4. Autoimmune Diseases

Therapy: Hematopoietic stem cell transplantation (HSCT) Mechanism: HSCT aims to "reset" the immune system by eradicating the faulty immune cells and regenerating a new, healthy immune system from transplanted stem cells. Clinical Evidence: HSCT has been used successfully in conditions like systemic lupus erythematosus (SLE) and multiple sclerosis (MS), showing significant improvements in disease progression and quality of life. [PMID34646275]

Hematopoietic Stem Cell Transplantation (HSCT): HSCT can reset the immune system by eradicating faulty immune cells and regenerating a healthy immune system. It has shown significant benefits in diseases like systemic lupus erythematosus (SLE) and multiple sclerosis (MS). [PMID23770628]

5. Autism

Therapy: MSCs Mechanism: MSCs may modulate neuroinflammation and support neural repair, potentially improving cognitive and behavioral functions in autism. Clinical Evidence: Preliminary studies and clinical trials have shown promising results in reducing symptoms and improving behavior in children with autism. [PMID24772244]

MSC Therapy: MSCs may modulate neuroinflammation and support neural repair, potentially improving cognitive and behavioral functions in children with autism. Preliminary studies and clinical trials have shown promising results. [PMID30842805]

6. Amyotrophic Lateral Sclerosis (ALS)

Therapy: MSCs and neural stem cells Mechanism: Stem cells may provide neurotrophic support, modulate the immune response, and promote neural repair in ALS. Clinical Evidence: Trials such as the NurOwn (using autologous MSCs) have shown safety and potential efficacy in slowing disease progression. [PMID35842587]

Neural Stem Cells and MSCs: Stem cells may provide neurotrophic support and promote neural repair in ALS. Trials, such as the NurOwn study, have shown potential in slowing disease progression. [PMID28926091]

7. Multiple Sclerosis (MS)

Therapy: HSCT and MSCs Mechanism: HSCT can reboot the immune system, while MSCs can modulate inflammation and promote neural repair. Clinical Evidence: Studies have shown significant improvements in disease activity and reduction in disability scores with HSCT. MSCs are also being explored for their potential to repair myelin and reduce inflammation. [PMID30039439, 37985645]

HSCT and MSCs: HSCT has shown significant improvements in disease activity and disability scores. MSCs are being explored for their potential to repair myelin and reduce inflammation. [PMID19513637]

8. Chronic Obstructive Pulmonary Disease (COPD)

Therapy: MSCs Mechanism: MSCs can reduce inflammation and promote the repair of lung tissue, potentially improving lung function. Clinical Evidence: Early-phase clinical trials have shown that MSC therapy can reduce inflammation and improve lung function in COPD patients.

MSCs: Early-phase clinical trials indicate that MSC therapy can reduce inflammation and improve lung function in COPD patients. [PMID35725505]

9. Macular Degeneration

Therapy: Retinal pigment epithelial (RPE) cells derived from stem cells Mechanism: Transplanted RPE cells can replace damaged cells in the retina, potentially restoring vision. [PMID38471273] Clinical Evidence: Trials using RPE cells derived from embryonic stem cells or induced pluripotent stem cells (iPSCs) have shown promising results in improving vision in patients with macular degeneration. [PMID36626080]

Retinal Pigment Epithelial (RPE) Cells: RPE cells derived from stem cells can replace damaged retinal cells, potentially restoring vision. Clinical trials have shown promising improvements in patients with macular degeneration. [PMID35835183]

10. Sickle Cell Disease

Therapy: HSCT Mechanism: HSCT replaces the defective hematopoietic stem cells with healthy ones from a donor, curing the disease. Clinical Evidence: HSCT has been shown to cure sickle cell disease in many patients, particularly those who receive transplants from matched sibling donors. [PMID35773052] HSCT has been shown to cure sickle cell disease, especially when using matched sibling donors.

11. Cerebral Palsy

MSCs and umbilical cord blood stem cells Mechanism: Stem cells may promote neuroprotection, reduce inflammation, and support neural repair, potentially improving motor function and cognitive outcomes. Clinical Evidence: Clinical trials have shown that stem cell therapy can improve motor function and cognitive outcomes in children with cerebral palsy. [PMID33853147] The authors showed recent 13 clinical trials using UC-MSCs for neurological disorders.

Umbilical Cord Blood Stem Cells and MSCs: Stem cell therapy may promote neuroprotection and support neural repair, improving motor function and cognitive outcomes in children with cerebral palsy. [PMID38261236]

12. Cancer

Cancer treatments with MSCs are also rapidly advancing as well as iPS and other genetic approaches. Weng 2021: "Therapeutic roles of mesenchymal stem cell-derived extracellular vesicles in cancer" [PMID34479611]

Traditional HSCT (bone marrow transplant) Mechanism: HSCT is used to restore bone marrow function after high-dose chemotherapy or radiation therapy used to treat cancers like leukemia and lymphoma. Clinical Evidence: HSCT is a well-established treatment for various hematologic cancers, improving survival rates and reducing relapse risk.

13. Intra-nasal delivery to the brain

The blood-brain barrier can be circumvented by a relatively simple intra-nasal delivery into the sinus cavity via a tube.

Mesenchymal stem cells sprayed into the rat noses migrated to the brain and survived for at least 6 months. [PMID21291297]

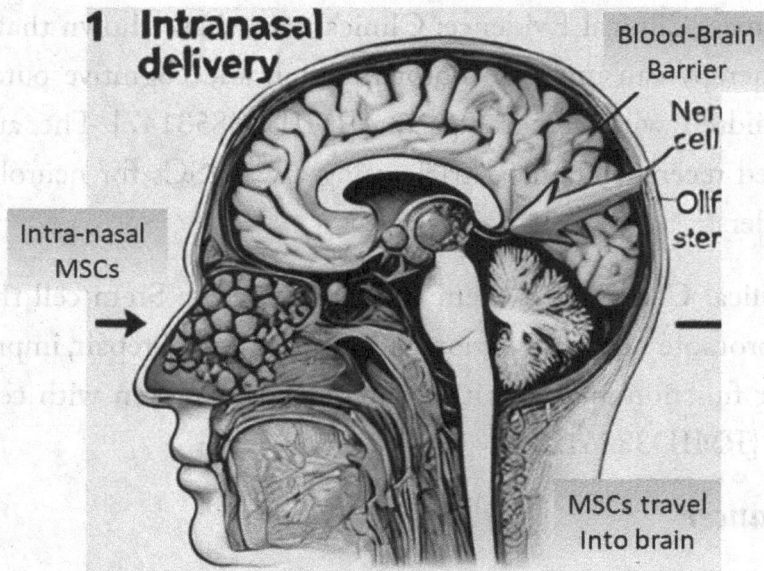

Fig.: 16 Schematic of MSC breaking into the blood brain barrier by intranasal delivery.

Fakiruddin 2018: "In this review, we first discuss the tumor-homing capacity of MSCs, its effect in tumor tropism, the different approach behind genetically-engineered MSCs, and the efficacy and safety of each agent delivered by these MSCs."

Reitz 2012: "Intranasal application of neural stem/progenitor cells (NSPCs) leads to a rapid, targeted migration of cells toward intracerebral gliomas. Intranasally administered NSPCs displayed a rapid, targeted tumor tropism with significant numbers of NSPCs accumulating specifically at the intracerebral glioma site within 6 hours after intranasal delivery" [PMID23283548]

Li 2018: "The local delivery of stem cells as therapeutic carriers against glioma has produced encouraging results, but encounters obstacles with regards to the repeatability and invasiveness of administration. Intranasal delivery of therapeutic stem cells could overcome these obstacles, among others, as a noninvasive and easily repeatable mode of administration." [PMID28895435]

13. Wound Care

Wounds, although superficial, involve an internal healing process. In older adults or individuals with conditions like diabetes, wounds can become chronic, leading to prolonged healing times that extend from days or weeks to months or years. Mesenchymal stem cells (MSCs) can play a significant role in wound healing by enhancing tissue regeneration, reducing inflammation, and promoting angiogenesis (formation of new blood vessels).

Amniotic Membranes

Amniotic Membranes were used in wound healing more than 100 years ago. These membranes have many regenerative benefits even in a dried and prepared form.

- **Rich in Growth Factors:** Amniotic membranes are rich in growth factors and cytokines that promote cell proliferation, differentiation, and tissue regeneration.

- **Anti-inflammatory and Antimicrobial:** They have natural anti-inflammatory and antimicrobial properties, reducing infection and inflammation at the wound site.

- **Biocompatibility:** Amniotic membranes are biocompatible and non-immunogenic, minimizing the risk of rejection and promoting integration with the host tissue.

Clinical Applications in Chronic Wounds: Used effectively in treating chronic wounds such as diabetic ulcers, venous stasis ulcers, and pressure sores, accelerating healing and reducing complications.

Burns and Surgical Wounds: Promotes rapid re-epithelialization, reducing scarring and improving functional and aesthetic outcomes.

How does this work?

Cell Proliferation: The presence of growth factors like EGF, TGF-β, and FGF promotes keratinocyte and fibroblast proliferation, essential for wound closure.

Anti-scarring: Amniotic membranes modulate fibroblast activity to prevent excessive scar tissue formation, leading to better healing outcomes. [PMID34909718]

As already mentioned in the introduction. Amniotic membranes provide a promising option for enhancing wound healing due to their rich content of bioactive molecules, anti-inflammatory properties, and biocompatibility. Their use in clinical settings for chronic and acute wounds has shown significant improvements in healing times and overall outcomes, making them a valuable tool in regenerative medicine.

Yang 2021: "Eleven randomized controlled trials with 816 participants total were identified in our review. Amniotic membrane treatment was more effective than conventional methods, silver sulfadiazine, and polyurethane membrane in treating burn wounds" [PMID33284236].

MSCs in Wound Healing

- Reduction of Inflammation: MSCs release anti-inflammatory cytokines that help r:educe chronic inflammation, a common issue in non-healing wounds.

- Angiogenesis: MSCs secrete growth factors like VEGF (vascular endothelial growth factor), promoting the formation of new blood vessels, which is crucial for delivering nutrients and oxygen to the wound site.

- Cell Proliferation and Differentiation: MSCs can differentiate into various cell types necessary for tissue repair, including fibroblasts, which are essential for ECM formation and wound contraction.

- Scar Reduction: MSCs modulate the immune response and ECM remodeling, reducing fibrosis and the formation of non-functional scar tissue.

Clinical Implications in Diabetic Ulcers: MSCs have shown promise in treating diabetic ulcers by accelerating healing and reducing complications. [PMID33995278]

Aging: In older adults, MSC therapy can enhance the body's natural healing processes, potentially reducing the incidence of chronic wounds.

Fig.17 shows a clinical patient report of a wound healing process (etiology: non-healing diabetic ulcer). The results speak for themselves, however this was not a controlled study and other healing modalities such as acupuncture and PEMF were also used. The patient was also under regular allopathic wound care.

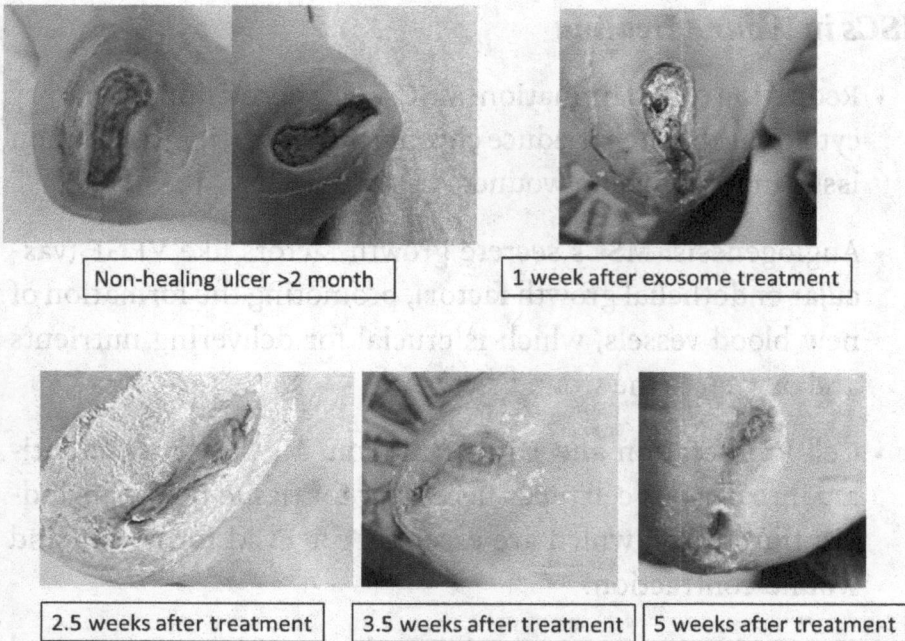

Fig.17: A non-healing ulcer that was injected with an exosome /secretome product. Shortly after injection the healing process appears starting to granulate and show signs of angiogenesis.

MSCs offer a promising approach to improving wound care, particularly in challenging cases such as diabetic ulcers and chronic wounds in older adults. Their ability to modulate inflammation, promote angiogenesis, and enhance tissue regeneration makes them a valuable tool in regenerative medicine for wound healing.

Conclusions - Internal Medicine

Stem cell therapies hold significant promise in treating a wide range of conditions within internal medicine. These therapies leverage the unique regenerative and immune-modulatory properties of stem cells to address the underlying causes of diseases and promote healing and recovery. While many of these therapies such as replacing pancreatic function in DM1 are still in the experimental or early clinical trial stages, the results so far are encouraging and suggest a transformative potential for stem cell-based treatments in the very near future.

Part V

Aging, Essence and the Philosophy of Stem Cells

The First Stem Cell

Living organisms had a beginning somewhere. The concept of the "first living cell" in the evolutionary history of life is an intriguing and complex discussion whether one believes in evolution or the creation model. While modern science does not precisely designate this first cell as a "stem cell" in the way we define stem cells today, it's possible to draw some parallels based on what we understand about early cellular life and the properties of stem cells.

Evolutionary Development of True Stem Cells

From Simple to Complex: As life evolved from single-cell organisms to multicellular ones, cells began to specialize and form more complex organisms. True stem cells emerged as part of this evolutionary trajectory, with specific stem cells evolving to maintain and regenerate tissues in multicellular organisms.

Role in Multicellularity: Stem cells in multicellular organisms are crucial for tissue growth, maintenance, and repair. Their evolution was a key factor in the development of organisms with specialized tissues and organs.

While the first cell was technically not a "stem cell" in the modern sense, its basic attributes of self-renewal and adaptability make it a conceptual precursor to what we now understand as stem cells in complex organisms. The evolution from these early cells to specialized cells and eventually to stem cells in multicellular organisms highlights the dynamic nature of life's evolution, with stem cells playing a crucial role in the development and complexity of life forms. Thus, while the first cell had stem-like qualities, the sophisticated functions of modern stem cells are a result of billions of years of evolutionary refinement.

The Definition of Life - Understanding a Cell

The Last Universal Common Ancestor (LUCA): Theoretical models and genetic studies suggest that the first cellular forms of life on Earth evolved from a common progenitor, known as the Last Universal Common Ancestor. This organism would have possessed the basic cellular machinery required for life, including the ability to replicate DNA, transcribe RNA, and translate proteins. The ability of self-renewal is generally said to be the most important characteristic of 'life'; however this is closely followed by metabolism and the cell membrane's function of selective permeability.

Self-renewal, metabolism, and selective permeability of cell membranes are all fundamental characteristics that define living organisms. Each of these features plays a crucial role in maintaining the basic functions necessary for life. Let's explore how each contributes to the broader understanding of what it means for a cell or an organism to be alive:

Key Features of Life

Reproduction and Renewal: One of the fundamental criteria for life is the ability to reproduce or make copies of oneself. Stem cells meet this criterion through their ability to self-renew, a process where they divide to produce more stem cells, maintaining their undifferentiated state.

Response to Stimuli: Living organisms are responsive to their environment. Stem cells have the ability to respond to signals in their environment, such as growth factors and cytokines, which dictate whether they remain quiescent, proliferate, or differentiate into specialized cells.

Growth and Differentiation: Another hallmark of life is the ability to grow and change. Stem cells embody this feature by not only supporting growth through replication but also demonstrating the potential for differentiation into a variety of cell types that contribute to the organism's development and repair.

DNA and Self-Renewal

Definition and Significance: Self-renewal is the ability of a cell to divide and give rise to more cells, which is particularly prominent in stem cells. This characteristic allows for the growth and maintenance of populations of cells within an organism and is essential for processes like development, healing, and tissue regeneration.

Stem cells hold a unique place in the realm of biology due to their distinctive DNA and inherent characteristics. Here's what sets them apart:

Pluripotency and Multipotency:

These cells, such as embryonic stem cells (ESCs) and induced pluripotent stem cells (iPSCs), have the potential to differentiate into almost any cell type in the body. Their DNA is marked by specific genetic and epigenetic signatures that maintain their undifferentiated state.

Genetic Signatures: Genes such as OCT4, SOX2, NANOG, and KLF4 are highly expressed in pluripotent stem cells, maintaining their undifferentiated state and capacity for self-renewal.

Surface Markers: Specific CD markers were discussed above. (CD73, CD90, and CD105 in mesenchymal stem cells are used to identify and isolate these cells).

DNA Methylation: Stem cells exhibit unique DNA methylation patterns, particularly at promoter regions of pluripotency genes. Hypomethylation in these regions keeps genes like OCT4 and NANOG active.

Histone Modifications: Specific histone modifications, such as H3K4me3 (tri-methylation of histone H3 at lysine 4), mark active promoters, while H3K27me3 (tri-methylation of histone H3 at lysine 27) marks repressed genes, maintaining the balance between self-renewal and differentiation.

Chromatin Structure: Stem cells have a more open and accessible chromatin structure, allowing for the flexible activation of genes required for pluripotency and differentiation.

Multipotent Stem Cells: Found in adult tissues (e.g., MSCs from bone marrow, adipose tissue), these can differentiate into a limited range of cell types related to their tissue of origin. Their DNA is slightly more restricted in potential compared to pluripotent stem cells.

Telomerase Activity: Stem cells exhibit high telomerase activity, which maintains the length of telomeres and allows them to divide extensively without undergoing the typical aging process that somatic cells experience. This contributes to their longevity and regenerative capacity. Beyond telomerase regulation, multiple genetic mechanisms, including the DNA damage response, CDK inhibitors, the Rb pathway, DNA methylation, and oncogene-induced senescence, contribute to limiting cell cycle divisions, ensuring cellular integrity and preventing uncontrolled proliferation. The telomerase activity and proliferative capacity of MSCs vary significantly based on their source. UC-MSCs typically exhibit the highest telomerase activity, followed by AD-MSCs and BM-MSCs. [PMID23380569]

Epigenetic Flexibility: Epigenetic Modifications: Stem cells possess a unique epigenetic landscape, characterized by a more open chromatin structure that allows for the expression of genes necessary for maintaining pluripotency or multipotency. These epigenetic marks can be reprogrammed during differentiation or dedifferentiation processes. Global DNA methylation patterns can change with age, leading to the repression of genes necessary for cell proliferation and promoting cellular senescence.

DNA Repair Mechanisms: Stem cells have robust DNA repair mechanisms to maintain genomic integrity over many cell divisions. This ensures that mutations are minimized, preserving their ability to generate healthy, differentiated cells.

Microenvironment and Niche Interaction: The microenvironment or niche where stem cells reside plays a critical role in regulating their function and maintaining their unique DNA characteristics. Signals from the niche help to maintain the balance between stem cell renewal and differentiation.

The unique properties of stem cell DNA are fundamental to their role in development, tissue maintenance, and regeneration. Understanding these properties not only provides insights into basic biological processes but also opens up potential therapeutic avenues for regenerative medicine, where harnessing the power of stem cells can lead to innovative treatments for a wide array of diseases and injuries.

Biological Role: In stem cells, self-renewal is balanced with differentiation. This balance ensures that organisms can develop diverse tissues while maintaining a pool of undifferentiated stem cells for future needs, embodying the dynamic and adaptive nature of biological systems.

Metabolism

Definition and Significance: Metabolism refers to the chemical reactions that occur within a cell or organism that are necessary for the maintenance of life. These reactions enable cells to grow, reproduce, maintain their structures, and respond to environmental changes.

Special Metabolism of Stem Cells

Stem cells possess a unique metabolic profile that supports their self-renewal and differentiation capabilities. Key aspects of their metabolism include:

Glycolysis Dominance: Stem cells primarily rely on glycolysis for energy production, even under normoxic conditions. This allows rapid ATP generation, which is crucial for maintaining stem cell functions.

Low Mitochondrial Activity: Stem cells have reduced oxidative phosphorylation. Stem cells exhibit lower mitochondrial activity and oxidative phosphorylation compared to differentiated cells. This minimizes the production of reactive oxygen species (ROS) and protects the stem cells from oxidative damage.

Metabolic Switching: During differentiation, stem cells switch from glycolysis to oxidative phosphorylation. This metabolic flexibility supports the diverse energy demands of different cell types as they mature.

Anabolic Pathways: High rates of nucleotide, protein, and lipid synthesis are essential for the rapid proliferation and self-renewal of stem cells.

Autophagy: Stem cells use autophagy to maintain cellular homeostasis by degrading and recycling damaged organelles and proteins, ensuring optimal function and longevity.

The special metabolism of stem cells, characterized by glycolysis dominance, low mitochondrial activity, and metabolic flexibility, is integral to their ability to self-renew and differentiate. These metabolic traits support their role in tissue maintenance and regeneration, making them a focal point in regenerative medicine research.

Biological Role: Metabolic processes are involved in energy production, synthesis of new molecules, and breakdown of waste products and toxins. Metabolism is not just a characteristic of individual cells but is also a critical component of how cells interact with and adapt to their environments.

Lipid Membranes in Stem Cells are high in Omega-3

The function of the cell membrane can be argued as the definition of a 'living cell'. Only when you control what goes in and out you create life and metabolism. And what would the DNA be without its nucleus and endoplasmic reticulum?

Definition and Significance: The cell membrane's selective permeability is essential for controlling the internal environment of a cell by regulating what substances can enter and exit. This feature is crucial for maintaining homeostasis within the cell. Stem cells have unique lipid membrane compositions that support their distinct functions. Through mechanisms like passive and active transport, cells can take in nutrients, expel waste, and communicate with their surroundings. The cell membrane's functionality is thus central to a cell's ability to thrive and function as part of a larger organism.

Key features of stem cell membranes

Lipid Rafts: Rich in omega-3, cholesterol and sphingolipids, lipid rafts organize cell signaling molecules, facilitating efficient signal transduction essential for stem cell maintenance and differentiation.

Function: These microdomains play a crucial role in maintaining stem cell pluripotency and guiding differentiation. The function of lipid rafts is highly dependent on omega-3.

Membrane Fluidity: Fatty Acid Composition: High levels of polyunsaturated fatty acids (PUFAs), including omega-3 fatty acids like DHA, enhance membrane fluidity, allowing dynamic cellular processes and adaptation to environmental changes.

Selective Permeability: Protein Channels and Transporters: Stem cell membranes possess specialized protein channels and transporters that regulate the selective uptake of nutrients, ions, and signaling molecules. This selective permeability is vital for maintaining the stem cell niche and facilitating communication with the surrounding environment.

Low ROS Production: The unique lipid composition especially due to omega-3 helps minimize the production of reactive oxygen species (ROS), protecting stem cells from oxidative stress and preserving their long-term functionality. [PMID31614433]

In summary, the special features of lipid membranes in stem cells, including the presence of lipid rafts, enhanced membrane fluidity, and selective permeability, are fundamental to their ability to self-renew, differentiate, and respond to environmental signals. These properties ensure the maintenance of stem cell integrity and functionality, highlighting their importance in tissue regeneration and repair.

An Integrative View

Complex organisms would certainly not be here without the function of stem cells. Renewal throughout life is important and necessary. Stem cells are called the 'essence of longevity' and will be discussed below.

Holistic Functionality: These characteristics are interconnected and contribute to a cell's ability to function as part of a complex living system. For example, a stem cell's ability to self-renew is influenced by its metabolic state and its ability to exchange materials with its surroundings through its selectively permeable membrane.

Life as a System: From a broader perspective, life can be viewed as a system in which these essential characteristics work together to create complex, dynamic, and adaptive organisms. The interplay between self-renewal, metabolism, and membrane permeability allows for the diverse forms and functions observed in the biological world.

The characteristics of self-renewal, metabolism, and selective permeability are foundational to our understanding of life. Each feature contributes uniquely to an organism's ability to sustain itself, adapt, and interact with its environment. In the context of cellular and molecular biology, appreciating these characteristics enhances our understanding of life's complexity and our approach to studying biological systems, from single cells to entire ecosystems.

The discussion around stem cells often intersects with broader philosophical and scientific debates about the definition of "life." Stem cells, due to their unique characteristics and roles in the development and maintenance of living organisms, provide a unique lens through which we can explore what it means to be "alive." Here's how the study and understanding of stem cells contribute to this discussion:

Philosophical and Ethical Dimensions

Potential for Life: Stem cells, especially embryonic stem cells, raise important ethical and philosophical questions about the potential for life. They have the capability to develop into a full organism under the right conditions, challenging and expanding our definitions of individual life and potential.

Identity and Change: The ability of stem cells to differentiate into different types of cells also dives into philosophical discussions about identity and what constitutes the essence of being. As stem cells differentiate, they transition from a state of pure potential to specialized entities, mirroring philosophical concepts of potentiality and actuality.

Scientific Implications

Origin of Life Research: Understanding how stem cells operate can provide insights into how life might have originated and evolved. For instance, learning how cells transitioned from simple replicative forms to complex systems capable of differentiation could mirror early evolutionary processes.

Artificial Life and Synthetic Biology: Research into stem cells aids in the development of synthetic biology and artificial life sciences, where researchers aim to recreate life-like properties in the lab. By manipulating stem cells or creating stem-cell-like entities, scientists explore the boundaries of what is technically alive.

Different Organs - Different Stem Cells

The concept of renewing every cell in the body varies significantly across different types of cells and tissues. Not all cells renew at the same rate, and some cells do not renew at all during a person's lifetime. Here's an overview of how long it typically takes for various cell types to renew, noting that these rates can be influenced by age, health, and environmental factors:

Cells with High Turnover Rates

- Skin Cells: The epidermis (outer layer of skin) renews itself roughly every 27 to 30 days.

- Red Blood Cells: These cells have a lifespan of about 120 days, after which they are replaced.

- Stomach Lining Cells: The cells lining the stomach renew every 2 to 9 days due to constant exposure to acidic conditions.

- Intestinal Cells (excluding the lining): These cells have a turnover rate of 4 to 5 days, some of the fastest in the body.

Cells with Moderate Turnover Rates

- Liver Cells: Liver cells turn over every 300-500 days, but this can vary based on liver health and injury.

- Endothelial Cells (lining blood vessels): These cells typically renew every few years, although this can be accelerated by physical activity or slowed down by vascular diseases.

Cells with Low or No Turnover Rates

- Cardiomyocytes (heart muscle cells): Some research suggests a very low turnover rate, with less than 1% of cardiomyocytes renewing annually. This rate decreases further with age.

- Neurons in the Central Nervous System: Many neurons in the brain do not regenerate under normal conditions and are considered permanent, lasting the individual's lifetime.

- Skeletal Muscle Cells: These cells regenerate at a very slow rate and primarily grow by increasing in size rather than quantity.

Age-Dependent Factors

Decreased Regeneration With Age: As individuals age, the overall capacity for cellular regeneration tends to decrease. This decline can contribute to the aging process and the onset of age-related diseases.

Stem Cell Exhaustion: The pool of stem cells, which are responsible for generating new cells, also diminishes with age, reducing the body's ability to repair and regenerate tissues effectively.

Special Stem Cells

Bone Cells: Osteocytes have a lifespan ranging from several years to decades, and bone remodeling is a continuous process that involves both the formation of new bone by osteoblasts and the resorption of old bone by osteoclasts.

Hair Follicles: Hair grows in cycles and each follicle can go through growth, transition, and resting phases before the hair falls out and the cycle restarts.

Hematopoietic Stem Cell Characteristics

Hematopoietic stem cells (HSCs) hold a special place in the process of immune cell renewal. In the bone marrow, they are crucial for the continuous renewal of blood cells throughout a person's life. These stem cells are responsible for producing all types of blood cells, including red blood cells, white blood cells, and platelets. Here's an overview of how hematopoietic stem cells are renewed and their special characteristics:

Self-Renewal: HSCs have the remarkable ability to replicate themselves through a process called self-renewal. This capability ensures a sustained pool of stem cells in the bone marrow to support lifelong blood cell production.

Multipotency: HSCs are multipotent, meaning they have the potential to differentiate into any type of blood cell depending on the body's needs. This versatility is critical for maintaining normal blood cell levels and responding to acute demands, such as in cases of injury or infection.

The Dynamics of Renewal and Differentiation

Balance Between Self-Renewal and Differentiation: HSCs must balance their self-renewal with the differentiation into specific blood cell lineages. This balance is regulated by a complex network of signaling pathways, transcription factors, and the bone marrow microenvironment.

- Bone Marrow Niche: The bone marrow niche is a specialized microenvironment that supports HSC maintenance, self-renewal, and differentiation. Cellular components (e.g., osteoblasts, endothelial cells) and extracellular matrix elements within the niche provide signals that help maintain HSC properties and regulate their activity.

- Extrinsic Signals: HSCs are regulated by extrinsic signals from the bone marrow niche, including cytokines, growth factors (such as stem cell factor and thrombopoietin), and interactions with the extracellular matrix and other niche cells.

- Intrinsic Factors: Intrinsic regulatory mechanisms within HSCs, including transcription factors like GATA-2, HOXB4, and Wnt/β-catenin pathways, play crucial roles in controlling self-renewal and differentiation.

Stem Cell Factor (SCF) / Kit Ligand

An example of an important cytokine is the Stem Cell Factor (SCF): Also known as Kit ligand or steel factor, is a cytokine that binds to the c-Kit receptor (CD117) on the surface of certain cells.

- SCF is crucial for the survival, proliferation, and differentiation of hematopoietic stem cells (HSCs), germ cells, and melanocytes. It plays a significant role in hematopoiesis (formation of blood cells), spermatogenesis, and melanogenesis (formation of melanin).

- Hematopoiesis: SCF is essential for the maintenance and expansion of hematopoietic stem cells in the bone marrow. It supports the early stages of blood cell development and ensures the continuous replenishment of blood cells.

- Spermatogenesis in Germ Cells: SCF is involved in the development of germ cells, playing a critical role in spermatogenesis by promoting the survival and proliferation of spermatogonial stem cells.

- Melanogenesis: SCF promotes the development and survival of melanocytes, which are responsible for the production of melanin. This function is important for pigmentation of the skin, hair, and eyes.

- Clinical Relevance and Therapeutic Potential: SCF has been investigated for its potential in treating conditions such as anemia, bone marrow failure, and certain types of infertility. Its role in stem cell mobilization makes it a candidate for enhancing stem cell transplants.

- Cancer Research: Abnormalities in SCF/c-Kit signaling are implicated in various cancers, including gastrointestinal stromal tumors (GISTs) and certain leukemias, making it a target for cancer therapies.

Stem Cell Factor (SCF) is a vital cytokine with broad implications in hematopoiesis, reproductive health, and pigmentation. Its therapeutic potential is being explored in various medical fields, highlighting its importance in both normal physiology and disease contexts.

Clinical Implications for HSCs

As research will zero into the targeted stem cell renewal of specific organs the bone marrow is certainly of prime focus.

Bone Marrow Transplants: HSCs are used therapeutically in bone marrow transplants for treating various hematological disorders, such as leukemia, lymphoma, and multiple myeloma. The ability of transplanted HSCs to reconstitute the entire hematopoietic system is a cornerstone of hematopoietic stem cell therapy.

Regenerative Medicine: Research continues to explore ways to expand HSCs in vitro while maintaining their multipotency, which could potentially increase the availability and efficacy of treatments for blood-related diseases.

Aging and HSC Function: As individuals age, HSCs tend to exhibit a bias towards producing certain lineages of blood cells, particularly myeloid cells, which can contribute to an increased risk of disorders such as myelodysplastic syndromes and anemia.

Disease Associations: Mutations and dysregulation in HSC function can lead to hematological malignancies. Understanding these processes is key to developing targeted therapies.

So, hematopoietic stem cells from bone marrow play a critical role in lifelong blood cell production through their unique capacities for self-renewal and differentiation. Ongoing research aims to better understand and harness these properties for therapeutic applications, improving outcomes in hematological treatments and regenerative medicine.

In summary, the rate of cell renewal varies widely depending on the cell type and is significantly affected by aging. Some cells have a high turnover rate and renew every few days, while others last a lifetime without replacement. This variability is crucial for understanding different health conditions and the body's response to injury and disease.

The first stem cell is special

Research on the "primordial stem cell" is interdisciplinary, involving developmental biology, genetics, molecular biology, and bioinformatics to unravel the complexities of early stem cell development.

Key areas of focus include:

- Embryonic Development: Studying the zygote and early embryonic stages to trace the lineage and characteristics of the first stem cells.

- Molecular Pathways: Investigating the signaling pathways and gene expression profiles that regulate stem cell pluripotency and differentiation.

- Epigenetic Regulation: Understanding how epigenetic modifications influence stem cell fate and maintain their totipotent state.

- Stem Cell Niches: Exploring the microenvironments that support and regulate the first stem cells in the early embryo.

Autopoiesis and Self-Replication: The first cell would need the capability to maintain and replicate itself, which is a fundamental property of life. This involves processes such as cell membrane formation, energy production, and the replication of genetic material.

Basic Properties: Like stem cells, the first cell would have had the ability to self-renew (replicate) and possibly the potential to give rise to more specialized forms (differentiate), as life became more complex. In this sense, the first cell might be considered a primordial form of a stem cell due to its fundamental capabilities.

Flexibility and Adaptation: Early cells had to be adaptable to survive in the harsh conditions of early Earth. This adaptability can be likened to how modern stem cells can differentiate based on their environment and signals they receive, a necessary trait for evolving into more complex multicellular organisms.

In conclusion, Stem cells, through their intrinsic properties and capabilities, contribute significantly to the ongoing discourse on what constitutes life. Their study not only advances our understanding of biological life's complexity but also pushes the boundaries of ethical, philosophical, and scientific exploration. As we continue to explore and manipulate the capabilities of stem cells, we may find that our definitions of life become more nuanced and perhaps even transformed.

Stem Cell Consciousness and the Quantum brain

We already established that stem cells carry special DNA characteristics. Could stem cells carry the "DNA of consciousness"? This question intertwines complex biological, philosophical, and neuroscientific considerations. From a scientific perspective, it's essential to clarify what could be the meaning of "DNA consciousness" and how this concept might relate to the function and genetics of stem cells.

Understanding Consciousness and DNA

Consciousness: Generally refers to the state of being aware of and able to think, feel, and respond to the environment. Consciousness involves cognition, awareness, perception, and subjective experience.

DNA: Deoxyribonucleic acid (DNA) carries genetic instructions used in the growth, development, functioning, and reproduction of all known organisms and many viruses. DNA sequences code for proteins, which are the molecular machines and structural components of cells.

DNA and Neural Development

While there currently is no evidence that DNA directly encodes for "consciousness", it contains the genetic instructions necessary for building the brain and nervous system, where consciousness is believed to reside. These instructions guide the development and function of neural circuits that underpin cognitive and perceptual processes associated with consciousness.

Role of Stem Cells

Neural Stem Cells: Stem cells, particularly neural stem cells, are critical for the development and maintenance of the brain. They generate neurons and glial cells which make up the complex circuitry of the nervous system.

Plasticity and Repair: In adults, neural stem cells are involved in neuroplasticity, which allows the brain to adapt to new information, experiences, and injuries. This plasticity is crucial for the brain's ability to encode and adapt functions that might be associated with aspects of consciousness.

Genetic Influence on Neural Functions

Gene Expression: The expression of genes involved in neural development and function can influence the structure and efficiency of neural networks, which might impact cognitive capacities and potentially aspects of consciousness.

Epigenetics: Modifications in gene expression that do not involve changes to the underlying DNA sequence (epigenetics) can also affect brain function and development, influenced by environmental factors, experiences, and neuronal activity.

Intranasal Delivery of MSCs and the Quantum Brain

Intranasal Delivery: As shown in PartIV, Intranasal administration allows MSCs to bypass the blood-brain barrier, providing direct access to the central nervous system.

Targeted Delivery: This method ensures that MSCs reach the brain more efficiently, enhancing their therapeutic potential for neurodegenerative diseases and brain injuries.

Potential Benefits for the Quantum Brain:

- Neuroprotection: MSCs can release neurotrophic factors that protect neurons from damage and support their survival.

- Anti-Inflammatory Effects: MSCs reduce neuroinflammation, which is crucial for maintaining cognitive functions and brain health.

- Regenerative Properties: MSCs promote the repair and regeneration of damaged neural tissues, potentially enhancing brain plasticity and function.

- Modulation of Brain Chemistry: MSCs might influence neurotransmitter systems and synaptic plasticity, contributing to improved neural communication and cognitive abilities.

How can MSCs assist the Quantum Processes:

- Quantum Coherence: Enhancing neural repair and function through MSCs might support theories that propose quantum coherence and entanglement in brain processes.

- Neural Synchronization: Improved cell signaling and neural network integration could facilitate complex brain functions and consciousness, aligning with quantum brain hypotheses.

- Enhanced Cognitive Function: By modulating brain chemistry and reducing inflammation, MSCs delivered intranasally could improve cognitive functions and potentially support the advanced processing proposed in quantum brain theories.

- Neuroregeneration: The regenerative properties of MSCs can aid in repairing neural circuits, crucial for maintaining the integrity of quantum processes in the brain.

Philosophical and Neuroscientific Perspectives

Consciousness as an Emergent Property: Many neuroscientists and philosophers argue that consciousness is an emergent property of the complex interactions within neural networks rather than something directly encoded in DNA.

Consciousness and Stem Cells: While stem cells contribute to the development and function of the brain, they do not inherently carry specific DNA sequences that can be described as encoding consciousness. Instead, they participate in the broader developmental processes that enable the brain to support conscious experience.

If "Stem cells" do bear the "DNA of consciousness" in a literal sense they are given to us for the purpose of physical and spiritual renewal and reconnecting us with the original source. While DNA provides the instructions necessary for brain development and function, consciousness is likely an emergent property of the complex interactions within the brain's neural networks. Stem cells play a crucial role in developing and maintaining these networks and in that sense they may encode at least a part of consciousness.

Stem Cell Origin and Consciousness

The idea that stem cells might be "closer to the original creation event" and therefore contain "more consciousness" blends metaphysical concepts with biological science. From a purely scientific perspective, stem cells are indeed primitive in the sense that they retain the capability to differentiate into various cell types and can self-renew to produce more stem cells. This versatility and potential make them fundamental to development and tissue regeneration. However, attributing qualities such as "consciousness" to cells, particularly on a comparative scale with other cells, moves beyond the boundaries of current scientific understanding and into philosophical or metaphysical interpretation.

As we discussed in this book, stem cells (omni-potent or pluri-potent) are special. They give life throughout life. They regenerate and sustain life. How do they accomplish this task? Much has to be done on understanding the life force behind these mechanisms. Again here the main points from a scientific perspective:

Pluripotency and Multipotency: Stem cells, especially embryonic stem cells, are pluripotent, meaning they have the potential to differentiate into any cell type in the body. Adult stem cells or somatic stem cells are generally multipotent, meaning their potential to differentiate is limited to cell types of a particular lineage.

Role in Development: Stem cells are critical during developmental stages for forming various tissues and organs. In adults, stem cells are involved in repairing and maintaining the structure of their tissue of origin.

Consciousness in Biological Terms

The Definition of human Consciousness is of much debate: In neuroscience, consciousness typically refers to an individual's awareness of their unique thoughts, memories, feelings, sensations, and environment. Consciousness is most commonly considered a function of the brain, particularly complex neural interactions in specific regions.

Neural Basis of Consciousness: Research suggests that consciousness arises from interconnected neural processes. Neurons, rather than stem cells, are the primary active agents in these processes, as they communicate through synapses and neural networks.

However where life and Consciousness exist in the body and how they connect is one of the mysteries of our creation. Chinese Medicine and other cultures have something more to say about this topic as discussed below.

Philosophical Considerations

Metaphysical Views: Some philosophical perspectives might view stem cells as more "fundamental" or "original" compared to differentiated cells, possibly attributing to them a greater connection to the origins of life or even a metaphysical quality like consciousness. However, these views do not reflect a scientific consensus but rather a philosophical or speculative interpretation.

Panpsychism: Some philosophies, like panpsychism, suggest that all matter could be imbued with a form of consciousness. Under such a view, one might argue that stem cells, as a more foundational form of biological matter, possess a form of consciousness. Again, this is a philosophical viewpoint, not a scientific one.

While scientifically, stem cells are not 'known' to contain or express consciousness they are definitely cells with the remarkable potential for differentiation and self-renewal. Attributes like consciousness are complex phenomena that, according to current understanding in neuroscience, arise from the interactions within networks of neurons, supported by but not directly arising from stem cells. Discussions about stem cells having more consciousness because they are closer to the "original creation event" are interesting from a metaphysical standpoint but remain outside the scope of empirical science.

Quantum Brain Theory and Omega-3

To conclude the discussion on consciousness and stem cells, it's important to explore the concept of the quantum brain and the unique role of omega-3 docosahexaenoic acid (DHA) in neural cell signaling throughout evolution.

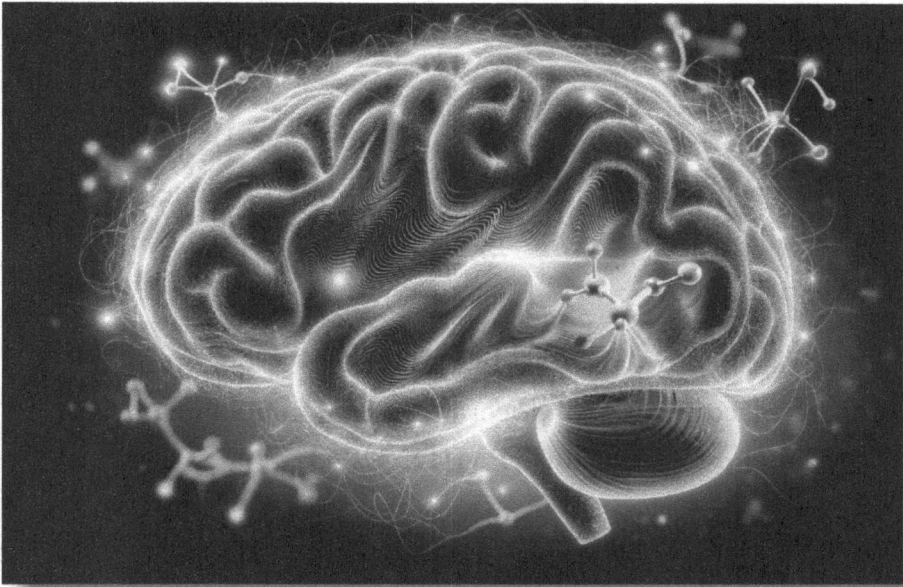

Fig.18: Omega-3 and MSCs influence your quantum brain capability through neural cell signaling and inflammatory control

Quantum Brain Theory:

Quantum Processes: The quantum brain theory suggests that quantum processes play a critical role in neural function and consciousness. This theory posits that the brain's computational power is enhanced by quantum coherence and entanglement, potentially explaining the complexity of human cognition and consciousness.

Microtubules and Quantum Computing: Some researchers propose that microtubules within neurons act as quantum processors, facilitating information processing at a quantum level. This quantum processing could contribute to the emergence of consciousness.

Role of DHA in Neural Cell Signaling:

Structural Importance: DHA, an omega-3 fatty acid, is a critical component of neuronal membranes, particularly in the brain. It maintains membrane fluidity, which is essential for proper cell signaling and function.

Evolutionary Perspective: Throughout evolution, DHA has been irreplaceable in neural development and function. Its unique chemical structure allows for efficient signaling and rapid transmission of neural impulses.

Crawford 2012 could not have said it any better: "A quantum theory for the irreplaceable role of docosahexaenoic acid in neural cell signaling throughout evolution" [PMID23206328]

Quantum Effects: The unique molecular structure of DHA may support quantum coherence in neural membranes, enhancing signal transmission and processing efficiency. This could be a key factor in the sophisticated neural functions associated with higher consciousness.

DHA Incorporation in Synaptic Membranes: Docosahexaenoic acid is crucial for the optimal functioning of synaptic membranes in the brain. Research has shown that synaptic membranes actively incorporate DHA with a high degree of selectivity. This selective incorporation is facilitated by π-electrons, which provide precise control over the energy of neural signals.

Mechanism: Synaptic membranes incorporate DHA through specific mechanisms that ensure its selective uptake and integration into the membrane lipid bilayer.

Role of π-Electrons: The π-electrons in DHA's structure play a critical role in its incorporation. These electrons allow for a high degree of selectivity and precision in the placement of DHA within the synaptic membrane.

Impact on Neural Signaling: The presence of DHA in synaptic membranes helps to precisely control the energy of neural signals. This precision is essential for efficient and accurate neurotransmission.

Membrane Fluidity: DHA contributes to the fluidity of the synaptic membrane, which is vital for the proper functioning of ion channels and receptors involved in neural communication. [PMID34400132]

Cognitive Function: The selective incorporation of DHA enhances cognitive functions, including learning and memory, by optimizing synaptic performance.

Neuroprotection: DHA provides neuroprotective effects, helping to prevent and repair damage to neural tissues. This is particularly important in neurodegenerative conditions. [PMID27866493]

In summary, DHA is selectively incorporated into synaptic membranes through mechanisms involving π-electrons, which ensure precise control over the energy of neural signals. This incorporation is crucial for maintaining membrane fluidity, enhancing cognitive function, and providing neuroprotection. Understanding these processes underscores the importance of DHA in brain health and highlights its potential in therapeutic applications for neurological disorders.

The Special Role of Omega-3 in Stem Cell Health and Their Niches

Omega-3 fatty acids, particularly docosahexaenoic acid (DHA), play a vital role in the health of stem cells and their niches. Here's how omega-3s contribute:

Structural and Functional Support- Membrane Fluidity and Integrity:

Omega-3 fatty acids are essential components of cell membranes, contributing to membrane fluidity and integrity. This is crucial for stem cells as it supports their structural stability and function.

Cell Signaling: DHA enhances cell signaling pathways, which are vital for stem cell differentiation and function. Proper signaling is essential for stem cells to respond to environmental cues and maintain their pluripotency or differentiate into specific cell types.

Anti-inflammatory Effects: Omega-3s have strong anti-inflammatory properties. Chronic inflammation can damage stem cells and their niches, impairing their function. By reducing inflammation, omega-3s create a more favorable environment for stem cell maintenance and activity.

Enhancing Stem Cell Niches and their Microenvironment:

The stem cell niche, the microenvironment where stem cells reside, is critical for their regulation. Omega-3s help modulate the niche by supporting the production of anti-inflammatory cytokines and growth factors that promote stem cell health and function.

Epigenetic Modifications: Omega-3 fatty acids can influence gene expression through epigenetic modifications. This regulation can enhance stem cell renewal and differentiation, contributing to tissue repair and regeneration.

Promoting Neurogenesis - Neural Stem Cells:

In the brain, DHA is particularly important for neural stem cells. It supports neurogenesis, the process by which new neurons are formed, which is essential for brain development, function, and repair.

Cognitive Function: Adequate levels of DHA are associated with better cognitive function and neuroprotection, highlighting the importance of omega-3s in maintaining the health of neural stem cells and their niches.

In conclusion, Omega-3 fatty acids, particularly DHA, play a crucial role in maintaining the health and function of stem cells and their niches. By supporting membrane integrity, reducing inflammation, and enhancing cell signaling and microenvironment regulation, omega-3s contribute significantly to the regenerative potential and overall health of stem cells. Ensuring adequate intake of omega-3s is vital for promoting stem cell health and their ability to repair and regenerate tissues throughout the body.

The intersection of quantum brain theory and the biological role of DHA in neural signaling provides a fascinating framework for understanding consciousness. By exploring these advanced concepts, we can better appreciate the complexity of the brain and the potential quantum mechanisms underlying our thoughts and awareness. This synthesis of quantum physics and neurobiology underscores the intricate and multifaceted nature of consciousness, offering new avenues for research and understanding in both science and medicine.

Essence (Jing 精)

The NeiJing says, "If the Sea of Marrow is abundant, vitality is good, the body feels light and agile, and the span of life will be long."

The connection between Traditional Chinese Medicine (TCM) concepts like the "Sea of Marrow" and "Jing" (精) and modern scientific understanding of stem cells and their niches is a fascinating example of how ancient wisdom can intersect with contemporary science. Exploring these parallels can provide a richer understanding of human health and the biological foundations of vitality and longevity. Here's an in-depth look at these concepts:

The Sea of Marrow in TCM

TCM Concept: In TCM, the "Sea of Marrow" is generally considered to fill the brain and spinal cord and connect to the bones. It is closely related to the central nervous system in modern anatomical terms. I propose a different interpretation here more related to overall contingency of the stem cells namely MSCs and HSCs resident within the bone marrow and other stem cell rich tissues. This makes more sense when discussing health and longevity.

Health Implications: According to TCM, the Sea of Marrow is crucial for cognitive functions, bone health, and overall vitality. A well-nourished Sea of Marrow is believed to contribute to a long and healthy life, mental clarity, and agility.

Jing (精) and Its Modern Parallels

In Traditional Chinese Medicine (TCM), Jing (精), often translated as "essence," is a fundamental concept that represents a deep, underlying basis of vitality. Jing is considered one of the three treasures in TCM, along with Qi (气, vital energy) and Shen (⊠, spirit or mind), and is crucial for health and longevity. Jing is categorized into two types: prenatal Jing (先天之精) and postnatal Jing (后天之精). Understanding both can provide insight into the holistic view of health and development in TCM.

TCM Concept: Jing or "essence," is considered a fundamental substance in TCM, representing stored energy that supports growth, reproduction, and development. Jing is believed to be inherited from one's parents and consumed gradually throughout life.

Connection to Stem Cells:

Conceptually, Jing shares similarities with the role of stem cells and their niches. Both are crucial for development, regeneration, and aging. Just as Jing is considered a determinant of vitality and resistance to disease, stem cells are essential for tissue regeneration and overall health.

Two distinct aspects of Jing are important. Epigenetics and parental genetics matters when it comes to your stem cell contingency but you also have to take good care of your stem cell longevity.

Prenatal Jing (先天之精)

Prenatal Jing is inherited from one's parents at conception. It is stored in the kidneys and is considered a fixed quantity that dictates one's constitutional strength, vitality, and potential lifespan.

- Characteristics: Prenatal Jing is the essence that determines one's basic constitution, strength, and vitality. It is analogous to genetic inheritance in Western medicine, influencing an individual's susceptibility to certain diseases and their overall health.

- Function: It governs growth, reproduction, and development. Major life changes such as puberty and menopause are considered manifestations of the fluctuations in prenatal Jing.

Conservation: In TCM, conserving prenatal Jing is crucial, as its depletion is thought to directly correlate with the aging process and general decline in physical health. Practices such as Tai Chi, Qigong, meditation, and adhering to dietary recommendations are advised to preserve prenatal Jing.

Postnatal Jing (后天之精)

Postnatal Jing is derived from food and air after birth through the processes of digestion and respiration, which are governed by the spleen and lungs, respectively.

- Characteristics: Unlike the fixed nature of prenatal Jing, postnatal Jing can be replenished and is influenced by lifestyle choices. It supports and replenishes prenatal Jing.

- Function: It plays a crucial role in fueling the body's day-to-day functions and contributes to the nourishment and maintenance of the body's tissues.

- Enhancement: A balanced diet, regular exercise, stress management, and healthy lifestyle choices are key to enhancing postnatal Jing.

Interrelationship and Health Implications

Balance and Support: Postnatal Jing supports and nourishes prenatal Jing. If postnatal Jing is abundant due to a healthy lifestyle, it can significantly reduce the rate at which prenatal Jing is consumed. This interrelationship highlights the TCM belief in the power of lifestyle modifications to affect one's health and longevity profoundly.

Health Practices: TCM practitioners often focus on dietary advice, herbal prescriptions, and Qi-gong exercises to strengthen the spleen and kidney functions, thereby enhancing the production and conservation of Jing.

Modern Interpretation

While the concepts of prenatal and postnatal Jing do not have direct equivalents in Western medicine, they broadly relate to genetic inheritance and environmental/lifestyle factors that influence health. Modern interpretations could view prenatal Jing as related to genetic predispositions and congenital conditions, whereas postnatal Jing could be analogous to factors influenced by diet, environment, and lifestyle.

In TCM, Jing is more than just a physical substance; it embodies a holistic approach to understanding the life force that drives growth, health, and aging. The balance and nurturing of Jing through integrated practices underscore the TCM focus on preventive health and the belief that lifestyle choices play a significant role in shaping one's health outcomes. This approach encourages a proactive attitude towards health maintenance and longevity, emphasizing harmony and balance within the body's systems.

Integrating TCM and Modern Science

Holistic Health Approaches: TCM's holistic approach, emphasizing the balance and flow of life forces, can complement modern medicine's more mechanistic view. The idea that maintaining the "Sea of Marrow" can influence longevity and vitality mirrors current research into how stem cell niches affect aging and regenerative capacity.

Preventive Medicine: TCM focuses on preventive measures to conserve Jing and promote longevity, which parallels modern preventive medicine strategies that aim to maintain stem cell health through diet, exercise, and avoiding environmental toxins.

Research Opportunities: Exploring the biochemical or cellular bases of TCM concepts like Jing might open new avenues for understanding how the body's intrinsic properties contribute to health and how they might be preserved or enhanced through both traditional and modern therapeutic approaches.

Thus, linking concepts from TCM such as the Sea of Marrow and Jing with contemporary understanding of stem cells provides a unique perspective that bridges traditional wisdom and modern science. This synthesis not only enriches our understanding of human health and longevity but also highlights the potential for integrative approaches that leverage centuries of knowledge alongside cutting-edge research. By viewing the body's regenerative capacities through both ancient and modern lenses, we can appreciate the complex interactions that govern health and disease and explore new ways to promote well-being and longevity.

Implications for stem cell therapy

Epigenetics, parental genetics, and the care of stem cell longevity— are integral to understanding how various factors influence our health, development, and aging process from both a modern scientific and a traditional Chinese Medicine (TCM) perspective. This holistic approach allows us to see how inherited traits and lifestyle choices interact to affect our overall well-being.

Parental Genetics and 'The Jing'

Parental Genetics: In modern science, parental genetics refers to the DNA inherited from both parents. This genetic material sets the groundwork for numerous physical traits, health conditions, and potential diseases. In TCM, this is closely related to prenatal Jing, which is considered the essence inherited from one's parents at conception, impacting one's constitution, vitality, and longevity.

Role of Prenatal Jing: Prenatal Jing, much like genetic inheritance, determines an individual's baseline resilience and potential health challenges. It is finite and viewed as a reservoir that depletes over one's lifetime. The better the quality of prenatal Jing one inherits, the better one's baseline health and resistance to disease.

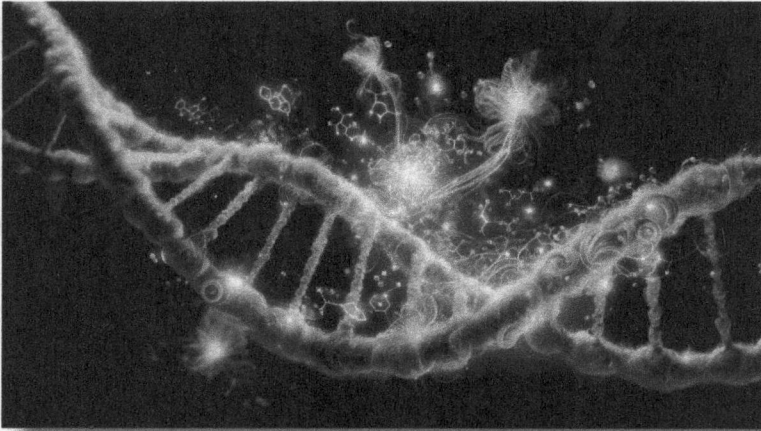

Fig.19: Parental Essence may dictate postnatal stem cell development through epigenetics

Epigenetics and Postnatal Jing

Epigenetics: Epigenetics involves changes in gene expression that do not alter the DNA sequence but still affect how cells read genes. This can be influenced by lifestyle factors such as diet, stress, and exposure to toxins. These changes can be temporary or, if occurring at critical times, may be long-lasting and even heritable.

Role of Postnatal Jing: Postnatal Jing, which is influenced by lifestyle choices and environmental factors, can be considered analogous to epigenetic changes. It is replenished and enhanced by good nutrition, healthy lifestyle choices, and effective stress management. Improving postnatal Jing can support and extend the lifespan and quality of the finite prenatal Jing.

Stem Cell Care for Longevity

Whether you are fortunate enough to have good Jing given to you at birth or are supplementing with modern stem cell sources, maintaining your health is crucial for preserving your stem cell niches. Practices from Chinese Medicine, including acupuncture, have been shown to support longevity and overall well-being. These traditional practices emphasize balance, proper diet, regular exercise, and stress management, all of which contribute to a healthy environment for stem cells, enhancing their ability to repair and regenerate tissues throughout life. Integrating these holistic approaches with modern advancements in stem cell therapy can maximize health benefits and promote longevity.

- Stem Cell Maintenance: Maintaining stem cell health involves protecting them from stress, environmental toxins, and inflammation, which can accelerate stem cell depletion and senescence. This is vital for ensuring that stem cells can continue to perform their roles in tissue regeneration and repair throughout life.

- Lifestyle Impacts: Lifestyle choices significantly impact stem cell health. A balanced diet rich in antioxidants, regular physical activity, adequate sleep, and stress reduction are all crucial for maintaining an environment conducive to stem cell longevity and functionality.

- Holistic Health Practices: Both modern holistic health practices and traditional methods like Qigong and Tai Ji focus on nurturing the body's inherent ability to heal and maintain itself, which can be seen as fostering both prenatal and postnatal Jing, and by extension, enhancing stem cell health.

Understanding the dual impact of genetics (prenatal Jing) and lifestyle (postnatal Jing) on health, as well as their relationship to stem cell functionality, offers a comprehensive approach to wellness that bridges ancient wisdom and modern science. This integrated perspective not only underscores the importance of genetic factors but also highlights the powerful role of epigenetic influences and daily health practices in shaping our biological health and longevity. The maintenance and care of stem cells through such holistic health practices ensure that we support our body's natural regenerative capabilities, promoting a longer, healthier life.

CONCLUSIONS: "Stem Cell Therapy in a Nutshell"

From the fundamental science behind stem cells to the practical applications in treating diseases, this book has explored the vast landscape of stem cell therapy, offering insights into both its potential and its challenges. Throughout the five parts, we've delved into the biological mechanisms of stem cells, their role in regenerative medicine, the implications of their use in treating autoimmune diseases, cardiovascular diseases, neurological conditions, and more. We've examined the ethical, philosophical, and regulatory issues surrounding stem cell research and therapy, integrating perspectives from traditional practices like Traditional Chinese Medicine to modern scientific approaches.

Delivering the complex topic of stem cell therapy in one book certainly constitutes a challenge, and many topics are missing or are only briefly mentioned. Please check the references for further reading. In summary, the author hopes to deliver an understanding of the importance of MSCs in reducing inflammation and scar reduction.

Here is a summary of what we have covered. Please refer to the table of contents to choose the special topics of your interest.

Part I: Introduction and Basics

The introduction sets the stage by emphasizing the shift from traditional symptom-based treatments to regenerative approaches. It highlights the unique potential of stem cell therapy to restore normal function by harnessing the body's innate healing capabilities. The introduction also provides a historical context and underscores the need for a balanced understanding of stem cell therapy's potential and limitations.

Part II: A Brief History of Stem Cell Discovery

This section traces the origins and milestones of stem cell research, focusing on the contributions of key figures like Dr. Arnold I. Caplan. It outlines the evolution of our understanding of mesenchymal stem cells (MSCs) and their application in regenerative medicine. Early discoveries, clinical trials, and the ethical considerations surrounding stem cell research are also discussed.

Part III: Scientific Background

In this part, we delve into the intricate science behind MSCs. It covers their ability to reduce inflammation through interleukins, modulate immune responses, and promote tissue regeneration. The section explores the mechanisms by which MSCs interact with their environment, including the role of microRNAs and chemokines in guiding differentiation and tissue repair. The scientific complexities and variabilities in MSC research are addressed, emphasizing the importance of standardized protocols and quality control. Here we also emphasize the importance of Omega-3 and how they assist the MSCs in their anti-inflammatory function.

Part IV: Applications and Case Studies

This section showcases the practical applications of MSC therapy across various medical fields. It provides case studies and clinical examples, demonstrating how MSCs are used to treat conditions like osteoarthritis, heart disease, autoimmune disorders, and more. The importance of measurable outcomes, such as WOMAC scores and MRI quantification, is highlighted to emphasize the efficacy of MSC treatments.

Part V: Stem Cells and Life

The final part of the book explores the philosophical and quantum perspectives on stem cells. It discusses the unique characteristics of stem cells that make them fundamental to life, such as their self-renewal capabilities and selective permeability. The section also touches on traditional Chinese medicine concepts, drawing parallels between ancient wisdom and modern stem cell science.

Furthermore, this book aims to bridge traditional and modern perspectives, emphasizing how advancements in stem cell research offer promising therapeutic potentials. Integrating knowledge from various disciplines, the text underscores the need for continued research, ethical considerations, and the integration of holistic health practices to maximize the benefits of stem cell therapy. The journey of understanding and utilizing stem cells is ongoing, and readers are encouraged to stay informed and engaged with emerging studies and breakthroughs in this transformative field.

Stem Cell Therapy - final thoughts

Stem cell therapy represents a frontier in medical science, offering revolutionary potential to heal and regenerate damaged tissues and organs. At its core, it utilizes the body's own building blocks to repair what has been lost or broken, potentially reversing the effects of diseases that were once considered untreatable. This therapy harnesses the power of stem cells, which are the body's raw materials — cells from which all other specialized cells are generated. Under the right conditions in the body or a laboratory, stem cells divide to form more cells called daughter cells. These daughter cells either become new stem cells (self-renewal) or become specialized cells (differentiation) with a more specific function, such as blood cells, brain cells, heart muscle cells, or bone cells. The promise of stem cell therapy lies not only in its ability to restore function and regenerate damaged tissues but also in its capacity to provide relief for chronic diseases by modulating immune system responses and reducing inflammation.

As we stand on the brink of what is a new era in regenerative medicine, it is clear that while the path forward is fraught with scientific, ethical, and regulatory challenges, the potential benefits of stem cell therapy make it a vital area of research. Continued exploration and innovation are essential to fully realize these benefits, as is a balanced discussion about the ethical implications of such profound biological manipulation. In essence, stem cell therapy encapsulates our greatest hopes for a future where the body's own cells can be guided to heal itself, offering hope for millions suffering from previously incurable ailments.

The author hopes this book has provided a foundational scientific understanding of the remarkable anti-inflammatory and regenerative capabilities of mesenchymal stem cells (MSCs). By exploring their roles in reducing inflammation, promoting tissue repair, and enhancing regenerative processes, we have highlighted the immense therapeutic potential of MSCs. This book aims to bridge the gap between complex scientific concepts and practical applications, empowering readers with knowledge about the benefits and current advancements in MSC therapy. For further reading and in-depth exploration, please refer to the references provided.

Appendix

How fast do organ-cells renew?

The renewal times of various organs or the turnover of their cells from fastest to slowest can provide a clear and useful reference. Below is a table outlining these renewal rates based on available data. Other than brain neurons, the heart and kidneys are among the least regenerative organs in the human body. Unlike tissues that can readily replace damaged cells, such as the skin or liver, the heart and kidneys have a limited ability to regenerate after injury. In the heart, cardiomyocytes, the cells responsible for heart contractions, have minimal capacity to proliferate, making recovery from damage, such as that caused by a heart attack, particularly challenging. Similarly, the kidneys, which are vital for filtering waste from the blood and maintaining fluid and electrolyte balance, have a restricted ability to regenerate nephrons, the functional units of the kidneys. Damage to these organs often leads to chronic conditions that require long-term management or interventions like dialysis or transplantation. The limited regenerative capacity of the heart and kidneys underscores the importance of advancing regenerative medicine and stem cell therapies to improve outcomes for patients with cardiovascular and renal diseases. Please note that these estimates can vary widely depending on individual health, age, and medical conditions:

Organ/Tissue	Turnover Time
Small intestine epithelium	2-4 days
Stomach	2-9 days
Blood Neutrophils	1-5 days
White blood cells Eosinophils	2-5 days
Gastrointestinal colon crypt cells	3-4 days
Cervix	6 days
Lungs alveoli	8 days
Tongue taste buds (rat)	10 days
Platelets	10 days
Bone osteoclasts	2 weeks
Intestine Paneth cells	20 days
Skin epidermis cells	10-30 days
Pancreas beta cells (rat)	20-50 days
Blood B cells (mouse)	4-7 weeks
Trachea	1-2 months
Hematopoietic stem cells	2 months
Sperm (male gametes)	2 months
Bone osteoblasts	3 months
Red blood cells	4 months
Liver hepatocyte cells	0.5-1 year
Fat cells	8 years
Cardiomyocytes	0.5-10% per year

Table 5: This table helps to understand the renewal times of different organs and tissues in the body, from those that regenerate quickly to those that do so more slowly.

A table of the age-related decline of stem cells in specific organs is provided below:

Tissue	Number of Stem Cells (Young Age)	Age-Related Loss	Number of Stem Cells (Old Age)
Hair Follicles	~100,000,000	Significant decline	~10,000,000
Gut Epithelium	~10,000,000,000	Moderate decline	~1,000,000,000
Heart	~1,000,000	Minimal decline	~100,000
Lung	~10,000,000	Moderate decline	~1,000,000
Bone Marrow	~1,000,000,000	Significant decline	~100,000,000
Liver	~100,000,000	Moderate decline	~10,000,000·
Kidney	~1,000,000	Moderate decline	~100,000
Brain	~100,000,000	Moderate decline	~10,000,000

Table 6: Approximate age-related stem cell numbers in various organ tissues

Notes: This table provides a broad overview of how frequently different organs and tissues renew their cells. It highlights the incredible diversity in regeneration capabilities across the human body, underscoring the complexity of biological systems and the influence of various factors on organ health and longevity. The number of stem cells in various tissues decreases with age, which affects the body's regenerative and repair capabilities. This decline is a crucial factor in the aging process and the development of age-related diseases. Understanding these changes can help develop targeted therapies to mitigate the effects of aging and improve health outcomes.

- Hair Follicles: Significant reduction from ~100 million to ~10 million.

- Gut Epithelium: Decline from ~10 billion to ~1 billion stem cells.

- Heart: Reduction from ~1 million to ~100,000 cardiac stem cells.

- Lung: Decline from ~10 million to ~1 million stem cells.

- Bone Marrow: Significant decrease from ~1 billion to ~100 million hematopoietic stem cells.

- Liver: Reduction from ~100 million to ~10 million hepatic stem cells.

- Kidney: Decline from ~1 million to ~100,000 renal stem cells.

- Brain: Moderate decline from ~100 million to ~10 million neural stem cells.

Variability: The renewal rates for some organs like the prostate, thyroid, and pancreas can vary significantly based on individual factors and available scientific data.

Age Factors: Renewal rates generally slow with age, and the capacity for regeneration can be compromised in older adults.

Disease Impact: Diseases can significantly alter the renewal capacities of these organs, either speeding up cell turnover as a compensatory mechanism or slowing it down due to damage or degeneration.

Dangers of Cortisone Injections

Cortisone injections are now known to cause significant bone and cartilage loss! Major side effects are:

- Skin discoloration or thinning: Injections near the surface of the skin can cause lightening of the skin color or thinning of the skin at the site of the injection.

- Elevated blood sugar levels: For people with diabetes, a cortisone injection can cause a temporary increase in blood sugar levels.

- Allergic reactions: Some people may experience an allergic reaction to the cortisone.

- Osteoporosis: Repeated cortisone injections can weaken bones (osteoporosis), particularly if given in the same location repeatedly.

- Tendon rupture: While rare, a cortisone injection near a tendon can lead to a rupture of the tendon.

- Nerve damage: If the needle touches a nerve during the injection, it can cause damage and pain.

- Steroid flare: This is a reaction to the injected cortisone that can result in increased pain and inflammation for up to 48 hours after the injection.

- Cartilage damage: Long-term, repeated injections into a joint can degrade cartilage, potentially accelerating joint damage.

Postmenopausal women suffered significant bone density loss in their hip after they were treated with an epidural steroid injection. [PMID 24404559, 34089066, 35524754]

"MRI measurements revealed thinning of knee cartilage in both groups by the end of the study. But loss of cartilage in the steroid group was significantly greater than in controls, with

the average change in cartilage thickness being -0.21 mm and -0.10 mm respectively." [PMID 28510679]

Joint Replacements: How effective?

The Efficacy and Comparison of artificial joint replacement with Stem Cell Therapies is a central point in modern stem cell therapy. What are the short and long term risks of surgery compared to stem cell therapy?

Does Knee Replacement surgery work?

Studies show that there is little to no benefit for long term joint replacement surgery:

- surgeries are at high risk for infections and even fdeath due to blood clots and anesthesia
- long recovery times and painful rehabilitation therapy
- patients still have pain associated with replaced joints
- limited range of motion and strength
- limited lifetime of artificial joints and the need for repeated surgery

In this controlled trial by Moseley 2002 involving patients with osteoarthritis of the knee, the outcomes after arthroscopic lavage or arthroscopic debridement were no better than those after a placebo procedure! [PMID 12110735]

Kirkley 2008: Arthroscopic surgery for osteoarthritis of the knee provides NO additional benefit to optimized physical and medical therapy. [PMID18784099]

Hip osteo-arthritis is among the most difficult to treat conditions due to the complex nature of the hip joint. Typically at a very advanced stage a hip replacement becomes necessary. Griffin 2018: "At 12 months after randomisation, mean iHOT-33 scores had improved from 39 to 58 for participants in the hip arthroscopy group, and from 35 to 49 in the personalized hip therapy group." [PMID29893223]

There is a limited number of meta-analyses comparing artificial joint replacement and stem cell therapy for osteoarthritis. Here's a brief overview based on current available research:

Artificial Joint Replacement - Efficacy: Proven to be highly effective in relieving pain and restoring function in severe osteoarthritis cases.

Risks: Includes surgical risks, potential for infection, and long recovery periods.

Stem Cell Therapy - Efficacy: Shows promise in reducing pain and improving joint function by regenerating cartilage, but results vary.

Risks: Generally lower than surgical interventions, but long-term efficacy and standardized protocols are still under investigation.

Need for Comparative Studies

The lack of comprehensive meta-analyses highlights the need for more rigorous, large-scale, and long-term studies to directly compare these two treatment modalities. Such research would provide clearer guidance on the efficacy, safety, and cost-effectiveness of stem cell therapy versus traditional joint replacement surgery for osteoarthritis.

Challenges in Insurance Coverage for Stem Cell Therapy

Regulatory Approval: FDA Approval Process: Insurance companies typically only cover FDA-approved treatments. The FDA approval process is stringent and time-consuming, involving multiple phases of clinical trials to ensure safety and efficacy. This can take decades, even for large biotech companies.

IND Process: Companies are undergoing Investigational New Drug (IND) applications to conduct clinical trials, but advancing to Phase 3 trials is challenging. Many Phase 3 trials for stem cell therapies have faced regulatory hurdles and have been blocked or delayed by the FDA.

Scientific and Economic Barriers: Variability in Results: Stem cell therapies can have variable outcomes based on the source of the stem cells, the condition being treated, and individual patient responses. This variability makes it harder to standardize treatments to meet regulatory requirements.

High Costs: Developing and manufacturing stem cell therapies is expensive. Without FDA approval, these treatments remain costly and are often considered experimental, making them less accessible and not covered by insurance. These high costs required by FDA phase trial regulations are carried by mostly small individual manufactures and institutions.

Ethical and Safety Concerns: The long-term safety and potential risks of stem cell therapies are still being studied. Concerns about the potential for tumor formation and immune reactions need to be thoroughly addressed in clinical trials.

Ethical Issues: The use of certain types of stem cells in the past, such as embryonic stem cells, raises ethical questions that complicate regulatory approval and public acceptance. As discussed, these tissues are not used in clinical applications and this discussion is mostly behind us.

While stem cell therapy has shown significant data in many clinical applications, its integration into mainstream medical practice and insurance coverage faces numerous challenges. These include the lengthy and rigorous FDA approval process, high development costs, variable clinical outcomes, and ongoing ethical and safety concerns. Continued research and successful clinical trials are crucial for overcoming these barriers and making stem cell therapies widely accessible and covered by insurance.

References:

FDA Approval Process: https://www.fda.gov/drugs/development-approval-process-drugs

Challenges in Stem Cell Therapy: [PMID29548515, 33615422, 35027497]

Insurance Coverage and Experimental Treatments in the US: "Insurance providers consider these orthobiologic treatments as experimental or speculative as long as there is no FDA approval" [PMID30466720]. Some countries such as Taiwan and Japan are moving stem cells into active clinical application: [PMID36498605, PMID34976978]

How effective is PRP?

Platelet-Rich Plasma (PRP) therapy is 'considered' a regenerative medicine technique wherein a concentration of platelets from a patient's own blood is injected into damaged tissues to promote healing. However, it is NOT a 'stem cell therapy' and PRP often has massive side effects and should not be confused with MSCs. The understanding of PRP's inflammatory and anti-inflammatory properties can be complex, so let's break it down:

Platelets and Inflammation: Platelets, by nature, play a role in both coagulation (blood clotting) and the body's inflammatory response. When tissues are injured, platelets release a variety of growth factors and cytokines. Some of these molecules can induce inflammation, which is a part of the body's natural healing process. Inflammation can help remove damaged cells and pathogens and prepare the tissue for repair.

Anti-Inflammatory Effects?: While platelets certainly initiate inflammation and many inflammatory markers such as IL-6 are present with this fraction of blood preparation, PRP also contains molecules that can reduce inflammation and pain. For instance, PRP has been shown to release anti-inflammatory cytokines and decrease the production of pro-inflammatory cytokines in certain settings. However the question remains if an individual (usually untested) blood sample has any such message.

Variability in PRP Preparations: Not all PRP is the same. Depending on how PRP is prepared, it can have different concentrations of platelets, white blood cells, and other components. For example, leukocyte-rich PRP (L-PRP) contains more white blood cells and might produce a stronger inflammatory response compared to leukocyte-poor PRP (P-PRP). The specific preparation and application can influence whether the PRP acts in a more inflammatory or anti-inflammatory manner.

Clinical Uses: PRP is used in various clinical settings, from orthopedic injuries to aesthetic medicine. The goal isn't necessarily to induce inflammation but to stimulate healing. In some cases, a short-term inflammatory response might be beneficial for healing, while in others, the anti-inflammatory and regenerative properties of PRP are more desired.

Research and Outcomes: The effectiveness of PRP is still a topic of research, and results can vary based on the condition being treated, the PRP preparation method, and individual patient factors. While there's evidence supporting the use of PRP for certain conditions, it's longer term effectiveness for all proposed applications has to be established. [PMID31775816]

Adverse Reactions: PRP injections of any kind and especially inter-osseous can have significant side effects of long term pain and trauma.

To summarize, PRP (platelet rich plasma) injections are prepared from the patient's OWN blood with a strict sterilized technique. After being centrifuged, the activated platelets are injected into the target area, releasing growth factors in the hope that they recruit and increase the bodies' own healing capacity. Although PRP contains a mixture of anti-inflammatory cytokines such as IL4,10 and TNFbeta; Platelets are by nature 'inflammatory' and they are not equal to stem cell therapy or MSCs.

Pre and Post-Care Guidelines for Stem Cell Therapy: Avoiding NSAIDs and Steroids

Effective pre and post-care is crucial for optimizing the outcomes of stem cell therapy. One of the key recommendations for patients undergoing this treatment is to avoid non-steroidal anti-inflammatory drugs (NSAIDs) and steroids. These medications can interfere with the healing processes that stem cell therapy aims to enhance.

Pre-Care Guidelines

Initial Assessment: A thorough medical assessment is necessary to understand the patient's overall health and specific needs.

Medication Review: Discuss all current medications with your healthcare provider to determine which ones need to be paused.

Discontinuation of NSAIDs and Steroids:

Timing: NSAIDs and steroids should be discontinued at least 1-2 weeks before the stem cell procedure, as advised by your healthcare provider.

Alternatives: Discuss alternative pain management options that do not interfere with the inflammatory processes crucial for stem cell efficacy.

Healthy Lifestyle:

Nutrition: Maintain a balanced diet rich in vitamins and minerals to support optimal stem cell function.

Hydration: Ensure adequate hydration to facilitate better cellular function and recovery.

Post-Care Guidelines

Inflammatory Response: NSAIDs and steroids can **inhibit** the necessary inflammatory response that stem cells rely on to promote healing and regeneration.

Duration: Continue to avoid these medications for at least 2-4 weeks post-treatment, or as directed by your healthcare provider.

Follow-Up Appointments: Attend all scheduled follow-up appointments to monitor progress and address any concerns promptly.

Adjustments: Your healthcare provider may adjust post-care instructions based on your response to the therapy.

Physical Activity: Gradually resume physical activities as advised. Avoid strenuous exercise immediately after the procedure to allow the stem cells to engraft and begin the healing process.

Rehabilitation: Engage in recommended physical therapy or rehabilitation exercises to support recovery and optimize outcomes.

Healthy Lifestyle Maintenance:

Diet and Hydration: Continue to follow a nutritious diet and stay well-hydrated to support overall health and recovery.

Supplements: Your healthcare provider may recommend specific supplements especially Omega-3, to enhance stem cell activity and recovery.

Avoiding NSAIDs and steroids before and after stem cell therapy is critical to ensuring the treatment's success. By following these pre and post-care guidelines, patients can maximize the therapeutic benefits of stem cell therapy and achieve better outcomes. Always consult with your healthcare provider for personalized care instructions tailored to your specific needs and conditions.

Scientific Terms and Glossary of Abbreviations in Stem Cell Terminology

Scientific Terms

Pluripotent: Ability of a stem cell to differentiate into any of the three germ layers: ectoderm, mesoderm, and endoderm.

Totipotent: Capacity of a cell to develop into a complete organism.

Multipotent: Ability to differentiate into a limited range of cell types.

Differentiation: Process by which a stem cell develops into a more specialized cell type.

Self-Renewal: Ability of a stem cell to undergo numerous cycles of cell division while maintaining an undifferentiated state.

Mesenchymal Stem Cells (MSCs): Stem cells that can differentiate into a variety of cell types including bone, cartilage, and fat cells.

Hematopoietic Stem Cells (HSCs): Stem cells that give rise to all the blood cell types.

Induced Pluripotent Stem Cells (iPSCs): Somatic cells reprogrammed to a pluripotent state by introducing specific genes.

Stem Cell Niche: The microenvironment where stem cells are found, which regulates their function.

Epigenetics: Study of changes in gene expression without altering the DNA sequence, often through chemical modifications.

Abbreviations

CD: Cluster of Differentiation (markers on cell surface)

DHA: Docosahexaenoic acid an omega-3 fatty acid

ECM: Extracellular Matrix

EPA: Eicosapentaenoic acid (EPA) an omega-3 fatty acid

ESCs: Embryonic Stem Cells

GFP: Green Fluorescent Protein

HGF (hepatocyte growth factor).

HSCs: Hematopoietic Stem Cells

IL: Interleukin

iPSCs: Induced Pluripotent Stem Cells

miRNA: micro RNA (type of non-coding RNA)

MSCs: Mesenchymal Stem Cells

NANOG: Homeobox Transcription Factor NANOG

OCT4: Octamer-Binding Transcription Factor 4

PCR: Polymerase Chain Reaction

PRP: Platelet-rich plasma

SOX2: SRY-Box Transcription Factor 2

TGF-β: Transforming Growth Factor-Beta

UC-MSC: umbilical cord MSC

VEGF: Vascular Endothelial Growth Factor

Sources

The literature indicates that different sources of mesenchymal stem cells (MSCs) have varying abundances and properties:

BM-MSCs (Bone Marrow-Derived Mesenchymal Stem Cells):

Definition: MSCs that are harvested from bone marrow. They have the ability to differentiate into various cell types, including bone, cartilage, and fat cells.

SVF (Stromal Vascular Fraction):

Definition: A heterogeneous cell population obtained from adipose (fat) tissue, which includes MSCs, endothelial cells, immune cells, and pericytes.

UC-MSCs (Umbilical Cord-Derived Mesenchymal Stem Cells):

Definition: MSCs derived from the Wharton's Jelly of the umbilical cord. They are highly proliferative and have robust immunomodulatory properties.

Wharton's Jelly (WJ): WJ in the umbilical cord is considered one of the richest sources of MSCs. It provides a high yield and has excellent proliferation potential. MSCs from WJ are primitive, exhibit robust immunomodulatory properties, and show significant regenerative potential. **Umbilical Cord Blood:** Contains a moderate number of MSCs but is more often used for hematopoietic stem cells. Advantages are non-invasive collection and good expansion capabilities.

Adipose Tissue: Adipose tissue is another abundant source of MSCs, often yielding higher quantities than bone marrow Advantages are easy to obtain through liposuction, high proliferative capacity, and significant potential for differentiation.

Bone Marrow (BM): BM has been the standard source for MSCs but typically provides a lower yield compared to WJ and adipose tissue. Advantages are well-characterized, with a long history of clinical use.

PRP: Blood is drawn from the patient and then placed into a centrifuge. Blood is spun through the centrifuge to separate the platelets and growth factors. This concentrated serum of platelets is then re-injected into the patient.

Sources, Characteristics, and Products in the Regenerative Market

Characteristics vs. Sources:

Characteristics	Umbilical Cord Matrix	Amniotic Matrix	PRP	Amniotic Fluid	Lipoaspirate	Bone Marrow Aspirate	Umbilical Cord Blood
Cytokines	✓		✓	✓	✓	✓	✓
Growth Factors	✓	✓	✓	✓	✓	✓	✓
Scaffolding Biomolecules	✓	✓					
Microvesicles & Exosomes	✓	✓					
Extracellular Matrix Biomolecules	✓	✓					
Native Cell Populations	✓				✓	✓	✓
Allogeneic	✓	✓		✓			✓
Autologous			✓		✓	✓	

Table 7: Comparative list of regenerative sources and their attributes

Additional References:

Dominici, M., et al. (2006). "Minimal criteria for defining multipotent mesenchymal stromal cells. The International Society for Cellular Therapy position statement." Cytotherapy. [PMID16923606]

Wang, H. S., et al. (2004). "Mesenchymal stem cells in the Wharton's jelly of the human umbilical cord." Stem Cells. [PMID25622293]

Gimble, J. M., et al. (2007). "Adipose-derived stem cells for regenerative medicine." Circulation Research. [PMID17495232]

Pittenger, M. F., et al. (1999). "Multilineage potential of adult human mesenchymal stem cells." Science. [PMID10102814]

Hyväri L, Vanhatupa S, Ojansivu M, Kelloniemi M, Pakarinen TK, Hupa L, Miettinen S. Heat Shock Protein 27 Is Involved in the Bioactive Glass Induced Osteogenic Response of Human Mesenchymal Stem Cells. Cells. 2023 Jan 5;12(2):224. [PMID36672159]

Li Z, MacDougald OA. Stem cell factor: the bridge between bone marrow adipocytes and hematopoietic cells. Haematologica. 2019 Sep;104(9):1689-1691. [PMID:31473604]

Boregowda SV, Krishnappa V, Phinney DG. Isolation of Mouse Bone Marrow Mesenchymal Stem Cells. Methods Mol Biol. 2016;1416:205-23. [PMID: 27236673]

Quirici N, Soligo D, Bossolasco P, Servida F, Lumini C, Deliliers GL. Isolation of bone marrow mesenchymal stem cells by anti-nerve growth factor receptor antibodies. Exp Hematol. 2002 Jul;30(7):783-91. [PMID: 12135677]

Plant based stem cells?

Plant-based stem cells cannot generate mesenchymal stem cells (MSCs) as found in mammals. MSCs are derived from mesodermal tissues in animals, and their properties are specific to animal physiology. However, plant stem cells can be cultured and produce a range of bioactive compounds beneficial for skincare and cosmetics.

Regarding human therapeutic applications, plant-based stem cells cannot be used to produce human MSCs or their secretomes due to fundamental biological differences between plant and animal cells. MSCs for therapeutic purposes must be sourced from human or animal tissues to ensure compatibility and efficacy.

Bioactive Compounds from Plant Stem Cells and Their Applications

Plant stem cells cannot generate MSCs, but they produce bioactive compounds beneficial for human applications, particularly in skincare and cosmetics. The types of bioactive compounds and their effects can vary depending on the plant source.

Common Bioactive Compounds:

- Antioxidants: Protect skin cells from oxidative stress and damage.

- Growth Factors: Stimulate cell renewal and repair.

- Anti-inflammatory Agents: Reduce inflammation and soothe skin.

- Polyphenols: Provide anti-aging benefits and protect against UV damage.

Comparison: Apple vs. Algae Stem Cells

Apple Stem Cells:

- Malus Domestica: Known for longevity properties.

- Bioactives: Antioxidants, phenolic compounds.

- Effects: Anti-aging, skin rejuvenation.

Algae Stem Cells:

- Marine Algae: Rich in minerals and vitamins.

- Bioactives: Polysaccharides, omega-3 fatty acids.

- Effects: Hydration, skin repair, anti-inflammatory.

Both apple and algae stem cells offer unique bioactive compounds beneficial for human skin health, but they differ in their specific properties and effects. Apple stem cells are more focused on anti-aging and rejuvenation, while algae stem cells provide hydration, repair, and anti-inflammatory benefits.

As of now, there are no reports of plant-based growth factors being directly injected into humans for therapeutic purposes. Plant-derived compounds are commonly used in topical formulations for skincare due to their beneficial properties like anti-aging, antioxidant, and anti-inflammatory effects. These bioactive compounds are generally applied externally rather than injected. The use of plant-based products in skincare and cosmetics continues to be popular, but the application is limited to topical treatments and not direct injections into human tissues.

References

All references cited with [PMID#] are direct citations listed on the pubmed index of the National Center for Biotechnology:

https://pubmed.ncbi.nlm.nih.gov/#

To obtain the full citation - Add the PMID # into the link above or perform an internet search.

Lastly Some Wisdoms:

Why don't stem cells use social media?

They prefer to divide and multiply in private!

What did one stem cell say to the other at the end of the day?

"I'm splitting. See you tomorrow!"

Why was the stem cell so good at solving puzzles?

It found itself in many different situations and could always adapt!

Why did the scientist talk to his stem cells?

He heard that a little feedback helps them differentiate better.

Why are stem cells the best listeners?

Because they know how to receive complex signals!

What do you call a nutty group of stem cells?

A cluster of differentiation!

Why did the stem cell become a chef?

It had a talent for whipping up organ dishes!

What kind of music do stem cells like?

Anything as long as it's not too specialized!

How do stem cells throw a party?

They start by splitting up and inviting all the tissues!

What did the stem cell say to the immune cell at the party?

"Don't mind me; I'm just here to blend in!"

www.ingramcontent.com/pod-product-compliance
Lightning Source LLC
Chambersburg PA
CBHW011158220326
41597CB00028BA/4705